Diagnostic Lymph Node Pathology

Diagnostic Lymph Node Pathology

Dennis H. Wright
Emeritus Professor of Pathology, Southampton University, Southampton, UK

Bruce J. Addis
Consultant Histopathologist, Department of Cellular Pathology, Southampton General Hospital, Southampton, UK

Anthony S.-Y. Leong
Medical Director, Hunter Area Pathology Service, Professor and Chair, Discipline of Anatomical Pathology, University of Newcastle, Australia

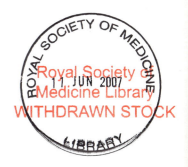
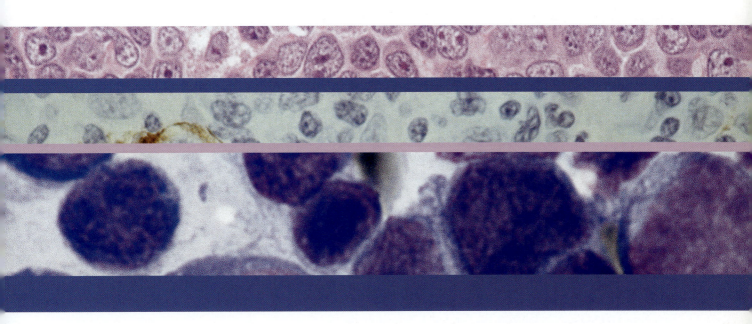

Hodder Arnold

A MEMBER OF THE HODDER HEADLINE GROUP

2006

First published in Great Britain in 2006 by
Hodder Arnold, an imprint of Hodder Education and a member of the Hodder Headline Group,
338 Euston Road, London NW1 3BH

http://www.hoddereducation.com

Distributed in the United States of America by
Oxford University Press Inc.,
198 Madison Avenue, New York, NY10016
Oxford is a registered trademark of Oxford University Press

British Library Cataloguing in Publication Data
A catalogue record for this book is available from the British Library

Library of Congress Cataloging-in-Publication Data
A catalog record for this book is available from the Library of Congress

ISBN-10   0 340 70609 0
ISBN-13   978 0 340 70609 1

1 2 3 4 5 6 7 8 9 10

Commissioning Editor: Joanna Koster
Project Editor: Heather Fyfe
Production Controller: Lindsay Smith
Cover Design: Sarah Rees

Typeset in 11/13 Goudy by Charon Tec Pvt. Ltd, Chennai, India
www.charontec.com
Printed and bound in Italy

What do you think about this book? Or any other Hodder Arnold title?
Please send your comments to www.hoddereducation.com

CONTENTS

PREFACE

Haematopathology has become the subject of specialist reporting in many countries in the developed world. This is seen as a necessary evolution and a consequence of the increasing complexity of the subject, the need for sophisticated ancillary investigations in some cases and the fundamental need for an accurate diagnosis on which to base further patient management. Nevertheless most lymph node biopsies will land on the desks of general pathologists who will need to make the judgement as to whether the pathology is that of a reactive or neoplastic process and whether referral is necessary. We have aimed this book at general pathologists and trainees, although we hope that dedicated haematopathologists may find some gems between its covers. In the light of our target readership we have placed our main emphasis on morphology rather than molecular techniques.

A number of authors have tried to base lymph node diagnosis on the low power structure of the node. While this is a good starting point it is not always helpful and can be misleading. For example, although an overall nodular pattern is characteristic of follicular lymphoma it can also be the dominant low power feature of mantle cell and marginal zone lymphomas. We would nevertheless emphasise the importance of both low power and high power morphologic examination based on good quality sections. It is wise to arrive at a diagnosis,

or differential diagnosis, based on morphology before ordering or embarking on the interpretation of immunohistochemical preparations. In the final analysis the morphology and immunohistochemistry should be compatible, and it is the concordance of these techniques that provides security of diagnosis.

We are aware of the time constraints facing pathologists and have aimed to make the basic information on entities easily accessible by presenting the clinical, morphological and immunohistochemical features of each disease together with illustrations in boxes. More detailed information is provided in the text.

Since we began writing this book we have seen a year on year growth of the proportion of lymph node biopsies received as needle biopsies. These are usually taken by radiologists using CT guidance. The most obvious value of this technique is in taking biopsies of deep seated lesions and thus avoiding the need for surgery. Most pathologists would probably wish that superficial nodes were obtained by whole lymph node biopsy. However, as clinicians realise that a definitive diagnosis can be obtained on a high proportion of superficial nodes using needle biopsies, this type of biopsy is likely to become more common in view of its ease of application and low morbidity. We have therefore included in the book a chapter specifically on the interpretation of needle biopsies.

1

HANDLING OF LYMPH NODE BIOPSIES, DIAGNOSTIC PROCEDURES AND RECOGNITION OF LYMPH NODE PATTERNS

TAKING AND HANDLING OF LYMPH NODE BIOPSIES

INTRODUCTION

Suboptimal techniques in the taking and handling of lymph node biopsies are probably the biggest obstacle to achieving a correct diagnosis. All concerned with this process should bear in mind that the objective of the biopsy is to achieve a timely and accurate diagnosis on which the subsequent management of the patient can be based. Feedback information at multidisciplinary team meetings is a valuable means of achieving and maintaining a high standard of lymph node biopsies. In the absence of such meetings, personal contact is needed to ensure that any shortcomings in the biopsy technique and handling of the specimen are rectified.

Lymph nodes should be selected for biopsy on the likelihood that they contain the pathological process. They should be dissected out whole, if possible, and with the capsule intact. Fragmented nodes may be more difficult to diagnose than intact nodes, depending on the pathological process involved. Traction artefacts are usually most severe when the biopsy tissue is very fibrotic or has to be taken from a confined space, such as the anterior mediastinum.

Needle biopsies are now more frequently used for the diagnosis of lymph node pathology. When possible, open lymph node biopsies should be used for superficial accessible lymph nodes; however, needle biopsies have a lower morbidity than open biopsies and are of particular value in sampling abdominal and retroperitoneal lymph nodes, avoiding the need for laparotomy. These biopsies are usually taken by radiologists using ultrasound or computed tomography (CT) guidance. Needle biopsies fixed quickly give good morphological preservation, which, together with immunohistochemistry, allows the precise identification of most common lymphomas. The technique may be less successful in the identification of non-neoplastic proliferations.

Fine needle aspiration biopsies have their greatest value in the separation of carcinoma from lymphoma and for the identification of recurrences or for staging.

The role of this technique for the primary diagnosis of lymphoma is limited and presents many pitfalls unless in the hand of an expert cytopathologist.

Logistics dictate that many laboratories receive their lymph node biopsies in fixative. In such cases, the volume of the fixative should be at least ten times that of the specimen. Whole lymph nodes should be sliced to allow rapid penetration of the fixative.

Ideally, lymph node biopsies should be received fresh in the laboratory immediately after excision. A slice taken from one end of the node can be gently touched on to clean glass slides, and air-dried and stained by one of the rapid Romanowsky techniques to provide a rapid cytological assessment. Pathologists experienced with this technique may give clinicians their provisional cytological diagnosis when appropriate. This technique is, however, most useful in determining the subsequent handling of the specimen in the laboratory. The slice of lymph node used to make the imprint preparation may be frozen for subsequent molecular investigation. It should not be used for histology, if this can be avoided, since the process of making imprint preparations often causes traction artefacts in the tissue.

Fresh tissue may be sent for cytogenetic analysis and/or flow cytometry in appropriate cases. Frozen sections may be cut for morphology and immunohistochemistry when indicated. One or more slices of the node should be placed in fixative overnight or longer for histology and immunohistochemistry. Needle biopsies require a similar period of fixation. Fortunately, for diagnostic purposes, a wide range of procedures, such as immunohistochemistry, polymerase chain reaction (PCR) for the detection of clonality, translocations, etc., and fluorescence *in-situ* hybridization (FISH) can be performed on fixed tissue.

BOX 1.1: Needle biopsies

- Tissue for histology and immunohistochemistry should be placed in isotonic fixative immediately. Do not allow to dry; do not leave in saline for long periods
- Allow at least 12 hours for fixation in formalin
- Additional cores may be taken for cytogenetics, molecular analysis, etc.
- Cut multiple sections for immunohistochemistry at the same time as the sections for routine stains are cut. This avoids the waste of tissue associated with recutting the block

---

BOX 1.2: Fresh whole lymph node biopsies

Slice using clean sharp blade; use slices as follows:

- Imprint cytology (tissue used to make imprints should not be used for histology)
- Histology and immunohistochemistry. Place slices in fixative, if using formalin fix for 12 to 24 hours
- Fresh tissue slices may be used for:
  - Cytogenetics
  - Molecular analysis
  - Cell culture
  - Microbiology

BOX 1.3: Fixed whole lymph node biopsies

- Cut into 5 mm slices with a sharp scalpel as soon as possible after biopsy
- Place in fixative, at least ten times the volume of the specimen
- Leave in fixative for 12–24 hours, if formalin is the fixative
- Tissue for long-term storage should be blocked in paraffin after fixation, not left in fixative

---

PROCESSING, SECTIONING AND STAINING

Laboratories should maintain quality control of their reagents and equipment to ensure adequate processing, cutting, staining and immunohistochemistry. Cell morphology is important in haematopathology, and can easily be obscured or distorted by poor fixation, processing and sectioning. Section thickness has a marked influence on cytological and histological appearances. The optimum thickness is 3–5 μm.

Haematoxylin and eosin (H&E) is the stain most widely used in histopathology and is often the only one used in lymph node diagnosis. The Giemsa stain can add another dimension to haematopathology and, in much of mainland Europe, is the stain of choice for this subspeciality. The Giemsa stain highlights basophilia and eosinophilia, and this aids the identification of blast cells, plasma cells, eosinophils and mast cells. When using this technique, care must be taken with the quality of the Giemsa stain used and the pH of the reagents, otherwise a section stained uniformly pale blue, of little diagnostic value, is obtained. The periodic acid–Schiff (PAS) stain may be of value in haematopathology. It highlights intranuclear immunoglobulin M (IgM) inclusions (Dutcher bodies), basement membrane and ground substance, such as that seen around the blood vessels in angioimmunoblastic T-cell lymphoma. The reticulin stain can be of value in determining the overall structure of the lymph node, highlighting follicularity, sinus structure and blood vessels.

In some laboratories, all of the stains described above are used as a 'lymph node set'. However, there is now a tendency to move directly from the H&E section to immunohistochemistry, when the additional use of one or more of these stains could be of greater diagnostic value.

IMMUNOHISTOCHEMISTRY

With experience and good histological preparations, it is possible to diagnose many of the common lymphomas on morphology alone. However, in most practices, a substantial number of cases cannot be categorized precisely without the aid of immunohistochemistry. Even in biopsies that are diagnosable with reasonable certainty on morphology alone, such as diffuse large B-cell lymphoma, immunohistochemistry will often provide additional prognostic information. It has, therefore, become standard practice in many laboratories to perform confirmatory immunohistochemistry on all lymphoma biopsies. The cost of this is trivial when set against the need to obtain an accurate diagnosis and the expense of treatment. Unfortunately, in the developing world, where obtaining and maintaining antibodies is often difficult, and no costs are trivial, diagnostic immunohistochemistry is not widely practised.

In our experience, it is not uncommon to receive biopsies from pathologists who have made a reasonable morphological diagnosis but have been confused by the subsequent immunohistochemistry. To avoid this pitfall, pathologists should be aware of the staining characteristics of antibodies and the specificity of their reactivity. The laboratory should be subject to ongoing quality control. For most antibodies used in haematopathology, there will be internal controls within the tissues being investigated (reactive B- and T-cells, histiocytes, etc.). For antigens not commonly expressed within normal and reactive tissues, such as anaplastic large cell kinase 1 (ALK-1), external control

tissues are necessary. Beware the section that is uniformly blue; it usually indicates technique failure.

Immunohistochemical techniques have improved considerably in the past decade with the production of increased numbers of robust antibodies and the development of techniques for antigen retrieval.

IS IT A LYMPHOMA?

Large cell lymphomas may resemble other anaplastic neoplasms. The leucocyte common antigen (LCA, CD45) shows membrane expression in almost all lymphoid cells and has only rarely been reported in non-haematopoietic cells. LCA may be absent on precursor (lymphoblastic) B- or T-cell lymphomas. Anaplastic large cell lymphomas are also often LCA negative, as are classic Hodgkin/Reed–Sternberg cells. Anaplastic large cell lymphomas frequently express epithelial membrane antigen (EMA), which together with LCA negativity may suggest an epithelial neoplasm. EMA is, however, expressed on plasma cells and on the cells of a number of lymphomas. Most epithelial neoplasms (carcinomas) express low-molecular-weight cytokeratins. In the rare cases in which low-molecular-weight cytokeratins have been reported in lymphoma cells, this has usually been in the form of a paranuclear dot. The majority of malignant melanomas can be identified with antibodies to S100 protein and HMB45.

IS IT A B-CELL LYMPHOMA?

Immunoglobulins

B-Lymphocytes are defined by their ability to synthesize immunoglobulins, which should, therefore, provide the most reliable means of identifying these cells. In practice, they are not used for this purpose in most laboratories. The main reason for this is that plasma immunoglobulins cause diffusion artefacts, particularly in poorly fixed specimens, that are often confusing and obscure specific staining. Cells that appear positive for immunoglobulins owing to passive uptake usually show smooth cytoplasmic staining that is most intense at the cell membrane. Within the node, these cells often occur in broad bands corresponding to the advancing front of the fixative as it diffuses into the tissue. Immunoglobulin in synthetic cells often appears granular, owing to its accumulation within the endoplasmic reticulum, or as larger inclusions. Synthesized immunoglobulin also frequently manifests as paranuclear (Golgi) staining and as strong staining around the nucleus corresponding to immunoglobulin within the perinuclear space. IgM is synthesized by a large proportion of diffuse large B-cell lymphomas and, because of its large molecular size and relatively low concentration in the plasma, shows less diffusion artefact than other immunoglobulins.

In addition to their use as B-cell lineage markers, immunoglobulins can be used as clonality markers. Clonal (neoplastic) populations are monotypic (i.e. they express only one light chain). Monotypia may be obscured by a background population of reactive cells, which usually express kappa and lambda light chains in the ratio of two to one. In general, reactive cells show more intense staining for immunoglobulins than neoplastic cells.

Although light chain restriction can be reliably identified in cells expressing cytoplasmic immunoglobulin, it is difficult to identify surface light chains except in the best fixed tissues. For this reason, immunoglobulin cannot always be used as a reliable clonality marker of small B-cells in paraffin-embedded tissue.

Surface IgD can be recognized in well-fixed paraffin-embedded tissues. Reactive mantle cells are positive, as are most cases of small lymphocytic lymphoma (CLL/SLL) and mantle cell lymphoma.

CD20 (L26)

CD20 is a non-glycosylated phosphoprotein expressed on the membrane of B-cells. Although widely regarded as such, it is not a perfect B-cell marker because it is not expressed in the earliest stages of B-cell differentiation and is lost as the B-cell undergoes plasma cell change. It is, therefore, absent on many B-lymphoblastic lymphomas and plasmacytic tumours. Staining for CD20 should be on the cell membrane, cytoplasmic, nuclear and nucleolar staining are non-specific. Because it is a surface membrane antigen, CD20 is often most strongly stained in biopsies that show some degree of shrinkage artefact and may appear less strongly stained in well-fixed tissues, such as needle biopsies.

CD20 has rarely been reported on T-cell lymphomas. It is expressed on the epithelial cells of thymoma (beware when diagnosing mediastinal large B-cell lymphoma).

CD79a

CD79 is a heterodimeric glycoprotein signal transduction molecule that associates with membrane immunoglobulin. Antibodies to the α-chain of the molecule (CD79a) provide an almost perfect B-cell lineage marker because CD79a is expressed throughout B-cell differentiation. It should be noted, however, that 50 per cent of T-lymphoblastic lymphomas express CD79a.

Staining for CD79a is cytoplasmic and is strong on plasma cells. It is more strongly expressed on mantle cells than on germinal centre cells.

Other markers

Details of other markers of value in the diagnosis of B-cell lymphomas are given below.

CD5

CD5 is a membrane glycoprotein expressed on T-cells. It is also expressed more weakly on the B-cells of B-CLL/SLL and mantle cell lymphoma. A small proportion of diffuse large B-cell lymphomas are positive for CD5.

CD10

CD10 recognizes a surface neutral endopeptidase (zinc-dependent metalloproteinase). Within the lymphoid system, it is expressed on the cells of B-lymphoblastic lymphoma, some T-lymphoblastic lymphomas and the neoplastic cells of some angioimmunoblastic T-cell lymphomas. Follicle centre cells express CD10, as do most follicular lymphomas. Burkitt lymphoma cells are positive, as are a proportion of diffuse large B-cell lymphomas (presumed to be of follicle centre cell origin). Outside the lymphoid system, CD10 is expressed on many stromal and epithelial cells, providing a positive internal control in many biopsies.

CD23

CD23 is a membrane glycoprotein expressed on activated B-cells. It also acts as a low-affinity receptor for IgE. In reactive tissues, CD23 is expressed on a variable proportion of mantle and follicle centre cells and on follicular dendritic cells. It labels the cells of B-CLL/SLL and provides a useful marker for this disease. It does not label mantle cell lymphoma but, owing to its reactivity with follicular dendritic cells, it highlights the dispersed pattern of these cells that is characteristic of this neoplasm.

BCL-1 (cyclin D1)

The cyclin D1 gene on chromosome 11q13 is translocated in mantle cell lymphoma, leading to overexpression of cyclin D1. Positive staining for cyclin D1 is seen in the nucleus; cytoplasmic staining is artefactual. This provides a valuable marker for the diagnosis of mantle cell lymphoma. Endothelial cells provide a positive internal control for the stain.

Cyclin D1 expression may also be seen in hairy cell leukaemia and some plasma cell tumours.

BCL-2

BCL-2 protein is coded by a gene on chromosome 18q21 that is involved in the 14:18 translocation characteristic of follicular lymphomas. It is a mitochondrial membrane protein that regulates apoptosis. In reactive tissues, small B- and T-cells are positive for BCL-2, whereas follicle centre B-cells are negative. Since 85 per cent of follicular lymphomas are BCL-2 positive, this provides a useful means of distinguishing between reactive and neoplastic follicles.

BCL-2 expression in diffuse large B-cell lymphomas has been shown in some studies to be associated with a poor prognosis.

BCL-6

BCL-6 is a zinc finger transcriptional repressor coded for on chromosome 3q27. Specific staining is nuclear; cytoplasmic staining is artefactual. In normal and reactive lymphoid tissue, nuclear staining for BCL-6 is seen in follicle centres but not in prefollicular or post-follicular cells. Most follicular lymphomas are BCL-6 positive. Burkitt lymphoma cells are positive. A high proportion of diffuse large B-cell lymphomas express BCL-6 but the percentage of positive nuclei varies. Overexpression of BCL-6 may be due to translocations involving 3q27 (present in up to 30 per cent of diffuse large B-cell lymphoma) or mutations of the gene. BCL-6 positivity may be used to identify follicle centre cell origin or as a prognostic marker.

CD45RA

Antibodies to variants of the CD45 molecule (4KB5, MB1, MT2) have been used in the past as markers of B-cells, but have been superseded by the more reliable and specific antibodies CD20 and CD79a. MT2 has been used as a marker for the distinction between reactive and neoplastic follicles. Although largely replaced by staining for BCL-2, this antibody might be worth considering in equivocal cases.

IS IT A T-CELL LYMPHOMA?

Many B-cell lymphomas contain large numbers of T-cells; indeed, these may be the majority population, as in some follicular lymphomas and in T-cell/histiocyte-rich B-cell lymphomas. The majority of these reactive T-cells will be small lymphocytes.

T-cell receptor

The defining antigen of the T-cell should be the T-cell receptor molecule (αβ or γδ). However, the only anti-bodies available that can be used with paraffin-embedded tissues are to the T-cell receptor β-chain. These only recognize T-cells with the αβ-receptor, are fixation dependent and are not widely used.

CD3

The CD3 molecule is a complex of four distinct glyco-protein chains that associate with the T-cell receptor (TCR). It is only when the CD3/TCR complex is fully assembled that it is inserted into the cell membrane. CD3 may, therefore, be detected either within the cytoplasm or at the cell surface. Theoretically, it provides the most reliable T-cell lineage marker, although it is lost or very weakly expressed in 20–25 per cent of T-cell lymphomas.

CD5

CD5 is an excellent marker of T-cells and is expressed in most T-cell lymphomas. The much weaker reaction of B-CLL/SLL and mantle cell lymphoma with CD5 is unlikely to cause diagnostic confusion because these tumours also express CD20 and CD79a.

Other markers of T-cell lymphomas

CD1a

This reacts with cortical thymocytes but is of most value in the diagnosis of Langerhans cell histiocytosis.

CD4

This is a marker of helper/inducer T-cells and their neo-plasms. It is also present on histiocytes, which may make interpretation of sections difficult.

CD8

This is a marker of suppressor/cytotoxic T-cells and neo-plasms derived from them.

CD7

This is expressed by T-cells and most T-cell neoplasms.

CD43 (MT1)

Antibodies to CD43 recognize a membrane mucin known as sialophorin. Although once widely used as a T-cell marker, CD43 has broad reactivity to many cell types, including some B-cell lymphomas. It is a useful marker of undifferentiated granulocytic neoplasms.

CD45RO

This was once widely used as a T-cell marker but has a broad reactivity. It has been largely superseded by antibodies to CD3 and CD5.

Cytotoxic granule-associated proteins (TIA1, perforin and granzyme B)

These antigens are revealed as cytoplasmic granules. They are expressed by cytotoxic T-cells and some T-cell lymphomas (e.g. anaplastic large cell lymphoma and enteropathy-associated T-cell lymphomas).

IS IT A NATURAL KILLER (NK)- OR T/NK-CELL LYMPHOMA?

CD56

CD56 is a membrane glycoprotein and a member of the immunoglobulin superfamily. It was originally identified in brain and designated neuronal cell adhesion molecule (NCAM). CD56 is a marker for NK- and T/NK-cell neoplasms. It is expressed in a proportion of cases of acute myeloid leukaemia and is strongly expressed on most neuroectodermal tumours.

CD57

The CD57 antigen is a glycoprotein expressed on a variable proportion of peripheral blood lymphocytes, not all of which have NK-cell activity. Approximately half of these cells are NK-cells, the remainder being CD8-positive T-cells. Some T- and NK-cell neoplasms express CD57, however, less than 10 per cent of CD56 positive nasal type T/NK-cell neoplasms express this antigen.

Many of the CD4 T-cells found in germinal centres express CD57. CD4-positive CD57-positive T-cells rosette the popcorn cells of nodular lymphocyte-predominant Hodgkin lymphoma; this feature might be of value in differentiating these tumours from other types of Hodgkin lymphoma and T-cell/histiocyte-rich B-cell lymphoma.

CD57 is expressed on a wide range of non-haematopoietic neoplasms.

IS IT A PRECURSOR B- OR T-CELL LYMPHOMA?

Terminal deoxynucleotidyl transferase (TdT)

Terminal deoxynucleotidyl transferase is an intra-nuclear DNA polymerase that catalyses the addition of deoxynucleotidyl residues to DNA. It is in part responsible for creating diversity of antibodies or T-cell receptors in the early stages of B- or T-cell development. It, therefore, provides a marker for precursor B- or T-cell lymphomas. It is also expressed in cases of myeloid leukaemia in lymphoid blast crisis. In normal tissues, TdT positivity is seen in cortical thymocytes and in 1–2 per cent of bone marrow lymphocytes (2–7 per cent in neonates).

Nuclear staining indicates positivity; cytoplasmic staining is artefactual and of no diagnostic significance.

IS IT HODGKIN LYMPHOMA?

CD30

CD30 is a member of the tumour necrosis factor/nerve growth factor receptor family. CD30 expression is associated with activation. Immunochemically it is seen as membrane and/or paranuclear staining. Diffuse cytoplasmic staining, often associated with poor fixation, is of no significance. Scattered small parafollicular blast cells are labelled in reactive tissues. Strong uniform positivity is seen in most anaplastic large cell lymphomas. The majority of Hodgkin/Reed–Sternberg (H/RS) cells in classic types of Hodgkin lymphoma are positive. A variable proportion of cells in some large B- and T-cell lymphomas express CD30.

CD15

Antibodies to CD15 recognize a specific sugar sequence known as X hapten. It is expressed in the later stages of myeloid differentiation and strong staining of polymorphs usually provides a good internal control. H/RS cells of classic Hodgkin lymphoma express CD15 on the cell membrane and/or as a granular paranuclear aggregate in 70–80 per cent of cases. Weaker staining may be seen in a small proportion of B- and T-cell lymphomas, including anaplastic large cell lymphoma.

Many epithelial cells and carcinomas express CD15.

IS IT A HISTIOCYTIC OR DENDRITIC CELL PROLIFERATION?

CD21

This antibody recognizes the complement receptor C3d that acts as the B-cell receptor for Epstein–Barr virus (EBV). It is expressed by a range of B-cells but, in paraffin-embedded tissues, the strong reactivity is with follicular dendritic cells for which it is an excellent marker.

CD23

See above.

Lysozyme

Lysozyme is an enzyme (muramidase) produced at many mucosal surfaces. It is also a good marker for normal and neoplastic cells of the myelomonocytic series including mature histiocytes. In poorly fixed tissues, it often shows confusing diffusion artefacts.

CD68

CD68 is a glycosylated transmembrane protein involved in lysosomal trafficking. It is, therefore, expressed in all cells containing lysosomes. There are several good monoclonal antibodies to CD68 that react with different epitopes on the molecule and give different reactivities. Thus the antibody KP1 reacts with benign and neoplastic histiocytes as well as myeloid precursors, granulocytes and most acute myeloid leukaemias. Antibody PGM1 reacts with benign and neoplastic monocytes and histiocytes, but not with granulocytic cells or their precursors.

Many small B-cell lymphomas show dot positivity for CD68.

S100 proteins

S100 proteins are calcium-binding proteins originally identified in brain tissue. The designation S100 was given because these proteins are soluble in 100 per cent neutral ammonium sulphate. Their main value in haematopathology is as a marker for Langerhans cells and interdigitating reticulum cells.

They also label many neural tumours and the majority of malignant melanomas.

PROLIFERATION MARKER

Ki67

Ki67 is a large non-histone nucleoprotein expressed through all phases of the cell cycle except G0. Expression begins at the end of G1 and reaches a maximum in the mitotic phase of the cycle. Thus the intensity of the nuclear staining is often variable. The proliferation fraction, as determined by Ki67 labelling, may have prognostic significance and is often diagnostically helpful, for example, in the distinction between small B-cell lymphomas (1–15 per cent), diffuse large B-cell lymphomas (40–95 per cent) and Burkitt lymphoma (100 per cent).

MISCELLANEOUS

ALK-1

ALK-1 recognizes a tyrosine kinase that is overexpressed in 85 per cent of T/Null anaplastic large cell lymphomas as a result of t(2;5) in 90 per cent of cases and of variant translocations in the remainder. Those cases with t(2;5) translocation show cytoplasmic, nuclear and nucleolar staining with ALK-1, as a result of the activity of the native nucleophosmin. The variant translocations give cytoplasmic and/or membrane staining only.

A small number of diffuse large B-cell lymphomas express ALK. These tumours usually have plasmablastic features and lack expression of CD20, CD79a and CD30. Rare cases in this group show t(2;5), others show t(2;17) involving the clathrin gene. Reactivity with ALK-1 in the latter group shows characteristic granular cytoplasmic staining. Some inflammatory myoblastic tumours show translocations of the ALK gene and express cytoplasmic ALK.

DIAGNOSING THE 'UNDIAGNOSABLE' BIOPSY

Biopsies may be deemed undiagnosable for a number of reasons: they are too small, there is a severe crush/traction artefact, or there is extensive necrosis. In the past, such biopsies were categorized as inadequate and a repeat biopsy requested – a step that is not always clinically possible or desirable. With modern antigen retrieval techniques and immunohistochemistry, it is often possible to obtain useful information from such biopsies, and even to arrive at a conclusive diagnosis.

It is worth reiterating that the biopsies in which the diagnosis is most difficult to make are those subjected to poor fixation (poor-quality fixative, small volume of fixative, slow penetration of fixative due to tissue size, inadequate fixation time). That is to say, it is the handling of the biopsy after surgery that is at fault, rather than the taking of the biopsy.

In such biopsies, not only is the cytomorphology degraded but so are many immunohistochemical reactions. Two antibodies that are particularly useful in biopsies showing traction artefact are L26 (CD20) and Ki67. CD20 is a robust membrane antigen that will often be found to outline large B-cells in biopsies that in H&E-stained sections appear totally crushed. It may similarly identify B-cells in infarcted tissue. Ki67, a nuclear antigen, commonly shows a clear-cut labelling fraction in biopsies showing traction/crush artefact. The labelling fraction is useful in distinguishing between slowly proliferating (low-grade) and rapidly proliferating (high-grade) lymphomas.

WHERE TO BEGIN? RECOGNIZING LYMPH NODE PATTERNS

INTRODUCTION

An experienced haematopathologist is usually able to assign a lymph node biopsy to one or more possible diagnostic categories (reactive, neoplastic, small cell, large cell, mixed) on the initial reading of the histology. Confirmation and refinement of the diagnosis may then be made by more detailed morphological assessment, immunohistochemistry, molecular techniques, genetics, etc. It is wasteful of resources, and often difficult and sometimes misleading to attempt to make a diagnosis without having first placed the biopsy into one or more possible morphological subgroups. Ultimately, there should be no discrepancy between the morphology and the ancillary investigations. Pathologists lacking in experience in haematopathology may find this initial categorization of biopsies difficult, which can lead to misdirection of further investigations.

Attempts have been made to construct an algorithm that will lead the inexperienced to the correct diagnosis. We have found that the breadth and complexity of haematopathology makes it difficult to construct and use such algorithms. The following outlines some of the features to look for in lymph node biopsies in order to place them in a diagnostic category.

SINUS ARCHITECTURE

IS THE SINUS ARCHITECTURE INTACT, OR PARTIALLY OR COMPLETELY DESTROYED?

The sinus architecture is often best visualized in reticulin-stained preparations. An intact sinus structure is usually seen in reactive lymph nodes, whereas complete or partial destruction of the sinus architecture is usual in most lymphomas. Exceptions are leukaemias and lymphomas that have leukaemic manifestations (myeloid, CLL/SLL, lymphoblastic), which may infiltrate nodes, leaving much of the sinus structure intact.

PROMINENT SINUSES

ARE THE SINUSES VERY PROMINENT? WHAT CELLS DO THEY CONTAIN?

Sinus histiocytosis may be seen in a number of reactive and inflammatory lymphadenopathies, particularly those involving the mesenteric lymph nodes. Lipid-filled histiocytes may be seen in postlymphangiogram lymph nodes and in Whipple disease. A sinus pattern is characteristic of many cases of Langerhans cell histiocytosis and of Rosai–Dorfman disease.

Neoplasms that may give a prominent sinus pattern include metastatic non-lymphoid tumours, anaplastic large cell lymphoma and some cases of diffuse large B-cell lymphoma.

CAPSULE

IS THE CAPSULE THICKENED; DOES THE LYMPHOPROLIFERATION EXTEND INTO THE PERINODAL TISSUES?

Thickening of the capsule is common in reactive/inflammatory processes. It is characteristic of the nodular sclerosing subtype of Hodgkin lymphoma. Extension beyond the capsule is often seen in malignant lymphomas (e.g. follicular lymphoma, angioimmunoblastic T-cell lymphoma) but is less commonly seen in reactive/inflammatory processes.

REACTIVE FOLLICLES

ARE REACTIVE FOLLICLES PRESENT?

Reactive follicles are, of course, characteristic of most reactive/inflammatory lymph nodes. They may, however, be seen in a number of lymphomas (e.g. marginal zone lymphoma, interfollicular Hodgkin lymphoma) and in lymph nodes showing early/partial infiltration by lymphoma. Thus residual reactive germinal follicles may be seen in lymphoblastic lymphoma, CLL/SLL and mantle cell lymphoma.

OVERALL GROWTH PATTERN

IS THE GROWTH PATTERN FOLLICULAR/ NODULAR OR DIFFUSE?

Follicular lymphomas recapitulate much of the structure of reactive lymphoid follicles and have a follicular growth pattern. Mantle cell and marginal zone lymphomas surround and then colonize reactive follicles, frequently giving the node an overall nodular structure. Prominent proliferation centres in CLL/SLL may make the growth pattern appear nodular on low-power inspection. Hodgkin lymphoma of the nodular lymphocyte-predominant, lymphocyte-rich classical and nodular sclerosis subtypes have a nodular growth pattern.

In addition to follicular hyperplasia, a nodular growth pattern is characteristic of Castleman disease.

PARACORTEX

IS THE PARACORTEX EXPANDED? IF SO, BY WHAT CELLS?

Paracortical expansion is characteristic of some reactive lymphadenopathies and is associated with viral infections. It is seen in its most extreme form in infectious mononucleosis when the paracortex is expanded by B- and T-blasts. In dermatopathic lymphadenopathy the paracortex is expanded by pale-staining interdigitating reticulum cells.

MARGINAL ZONE

ARE THERE PROMINENT SINUSOIDAL, PARASINUSOIDAL OR PERIFOLLICULAR MONOCYTOID B-CELLS (CELLS WITH OVAL NUCLEI AND CLEAR CYTOPLASM)?

Monocytoid B-cell proliferation is characteristic of lymphadenopathy in human immunodeficiency virus (HIV) infection and in toxoplasmosis.

NECROSIS

DOES THE LYMPH NODE SHOW AREAS OF NECROSIS?

Caseous necrosis is characteristic of tuberculosis. Serpiginous areas of necrosis may be seen in cat scratch disease and in lymphogranuloma venereum. 'Normal' or neoplastic lymph nodes may undergo infarction. Areas of necrosis are relatively common in large cell lymphomas but rare in small cell lymphomas. When present in small cell lymphomas, necrosis usually indicates additional pathology such as virus infection. Angioinvasive lymphoproliferations, such as extranodal NK/T-cell lymphoma, nasal-type and lymphomatoid granulomatosis, usually show varying degrees of necrosis.

APOPTOSIS

DO MANY CELLS SHOW APOPTOSIS?

Apoptosis is a characteristic finding in reactive germinal centres. It is commonly seen in malignant lymphomas with a high growth fraction and is particularly prominent in Burkitt lymphoma. The apoptotic debris may be seen between viable cells or within macrophages. Apoptosis is a striking feature of Kikuchi–Fujimoto disease.

Apoptotic granulocytes may be seen in inflammatory conditions. If there is any doubt as to the nature of these bodies, they may be identified by immunohistochemistry using a granulocytic marker such as CD15.

GRANULOMAS

DOES THE LYMPH NODE CONTAIN EPITHELIOID CELL/GIANT CELL GRANULOMAS? ARE THESE WELL DEFINED? DO THEY SHOW NECROSIS?

Foreign material and infection may induce granulomatous inflammation in lymph nodes. Tuberculosis (necrotizing confluent granulomas) and sarcoidosis (non-necrotizing discrete granulomas) are among the most common causes of granulomatous lymphadenitis.

Epithelioid cell clusters, sometimes with giant cells, are frequently seen in Hodgkin lymphoma and some T-cell lymphomas (Lennert lymphoma). Large numbers of epithelioid cells in sheets or clusters may be seen in other lymphomas. They are often prominent in marginal zone lymphoma, T-cell histiocyte-rich B-cell lymphoma and anaplastic large cell lymphoma (lymphohistiocytic variant).

Lymph nodes from different anatomical sites show variation in their structure. Cervical lymph nodes exhibit the characteristic pattern of follicles, paracortex, medulla and sinuses. Axillary lymph nodes in their resting state appear as a rim of lymphoid tissue around a core of fat. In malignant lymphomas and other lymphoproliferations, this fat is colonized and may disappear completely. Mesenteric nodes have more prominent sinuses, and usually less conspicuous follicles and paracortex.

LYMPHOID FOLLICLES

These structures generate T-dependent antibody responses. They are the site at which the development of antibody diversity and isotype switching occurs. Primary follicles are composed of small B-cells, bearing surface immunoglobulin M (IgM) and IgD, and follicular dendritic cells. If a secondary follicle is sectioned at one pole, so as not to include the germinal centre, it will appear as a primary follicle. Secondary follicles have a germinal centre composed of blast cells (centroblasts) and their progeny (centrocytes). These cells show polarity, with the blast cells forming the dark zone (because of their deep cytoplasmic basophilia in Giemsa-stained preparations) and the centrocytes the light zone. The cells of the dark zone show numerous mitotic figures and have a high proliferation fraction; many may show features of apoptosis. Follicular polarity is usually better seen in lymphoid follicles at mucosal surfaces, such as the tonsil, than in lymph nodes.

Germinal centre B-cells do not express BCL-2 and are thus susceptible to apoptosis. Only those B-cells selected for good antibody affinity are allowed to re-express BCL-2 and survive. A high proportion of follicle centre B-cells undergo apoptosis and are ingested by macrophages within the centre (tingible body macrophages).

The germinal centre is surrounded by the mantle zone composed of small B-lymphocytes of the same phenotype as those seen in primary follicles. Marginal zone B-cells with clear cytoplasm may be seen outside the mantle zone. These are often seen in mesenteric nodes, but are usually inconspicuous at other sites. Lymphoid follicles contain a network of follicular dendritic cells (FDC). FDC capture and retain immune complexes on their surface for presentation to B- and T-cells. The nuclei of FDC are characteristic, often appearing binucleate or multinucleated. The dendritic processes are not identifiable in routinely stained sections but are often highlighted in sections stained for IgM, which labels immune complexes on the surface of the processes. Staining for CD21 and CD23 also highlights these processes. Involuting germinal centres often contain interstitial eosinophilic proteinaceous material. Plasma cells are sometimes seen in the germinal centres of reactive lymph nodes. Lymphoid follicles contain a variable number of small T-cells, many of which express CD3, CD4 and CD57.

PARACORTEX

The paracortex, deep to the follicles, is composed largely of T-cells with scattered B-cells. Depending on the reactive state of the node, there may be variable numbers of B- and T-blasts present. Characteristic high endothelial venules are seen within the paracortex. In these vessels, the endothelial cells appear cuboidal. Selectins expressed on these cells direct the traffic of lymphocytes from the blood into the lymph node. These small lymphocytes are often seen between the endothelial cells, or between them and the basement membrane.

Non-phagocytic antigen processing cells, known as interdigitating reticulum cells (IDRC), are present in the paracortex. These cells have numerous filament-ous cytoplasmic processes when seen in cell suspensions. It is the complex interdigitating of these processes between adjacent cells, as seen in electron micrographs, that gives them their name. IDRC have many similarities to Langerhans cells, but do not contain Birbeck granules. They are positive for S100 protein and HLA-DR. They have complex deeply clefted nuclei with small nucleoli. Scattered phagocytic histiocytes are also found in the paracortex.

Cells previously known as plasmacytoid T-cells are found in the paracortex in variable numbers. These were originally thought to be T-cells because of their reactivity with CD4 but this antigen is also expressed by cells of the monocyte lineage to which these cells

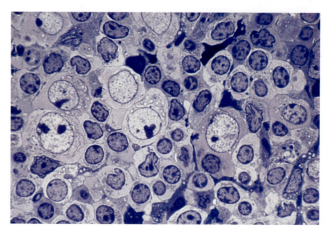

FIGURE 2.3 Plastic-embedded section of a reactive follicle showing centroblasts with visible nucleoli together with smaller centrocytes, a few of which show clefted nuclei.

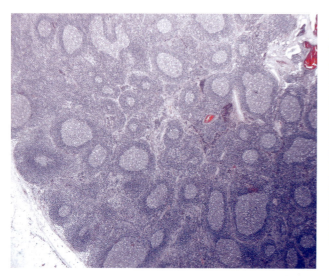

FIGURE 2.1 Low-power view of a reactive lymph node. Note the irregularity of size and shape of the reactive follicles, which have well-defined mantles. The subcapsular sinus and some medullary sinuses are recognizable.

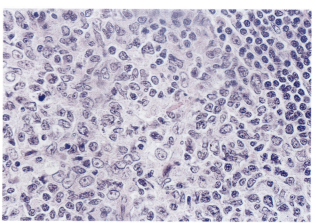

FIGURE 2.4 Regressing reactive germinal centre consisting mainly of centrocytes. The nuclei of several dendritic reticulum cells are present. These have oval nuclei with a well-defined nuclear membrane and a single eosinophilic nucleolus. These nuclei appear singly, in pairs or as small clusters.

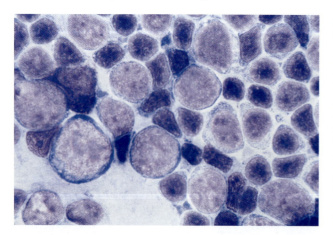

FIGURE 2.2 Imprint preparation of a reactive lymph node showing centroblasts with basophilic cytoplasm and visible nucleoli. The smaller lymphoid cells are a mixture of centrocytes and T-cells.

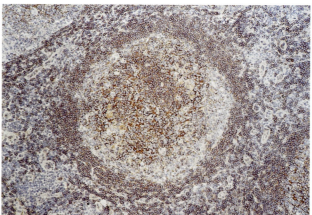

FIGURE 2.5 Reactive germinal follicle stained for immunoglobulin M (IgM). Note the positive staining of mantle cells and deposition of IgM, in the form of immune complexes, on follicular dendritic cells.

belong. They express CD68 and are now designated as plasmacytoid monocytes. Plasmacytoid monocytes may occur as single cells, small clusters or larger aggregates that may mimic follicle centres. The cells are of

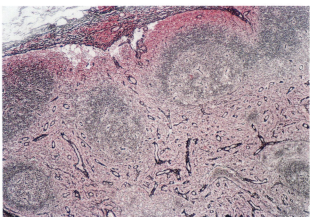

FIGURE 2.9 Reactive lymph node stained by the Gordon and Sweet method to show reticulin. Note the vascularity of the paracortex.

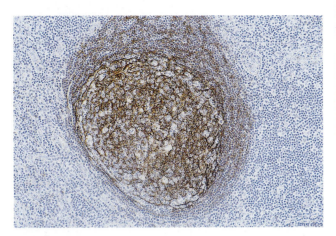

FIGURE 2.6 Reactive germinal follicle stained for CD21 to show follicular dendritic cells.

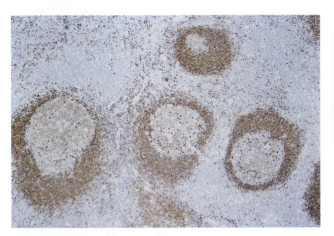

FIGURE 2.7 Reactive germinal follicles stained for CD79a. Note the well-defined, strongly stained mantle zones.

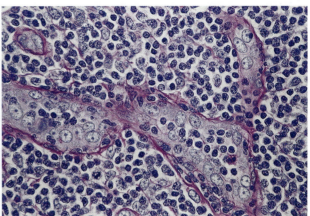

FIGURE 2.10 Paracortex of a reactive lymph node stained by the periodic acid–Schiff (PAS) technique. PAS-positive staining outlines a high endothelial venule containing many small lymphocytes in the lumen.

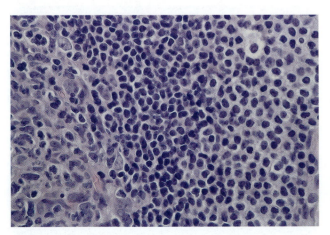

FIGURE 2.8 High-power view of a reactive germinal follicle showing the germinal centre cells (left), mantle cells (centre) and marginal zone cells with increased clear cytoplasm (right).

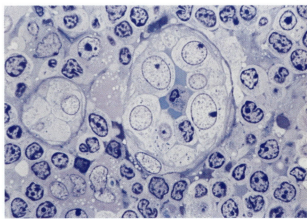

FIGURE 2.11 Plastic-embedded section from the paracortex of a reactive lymph node showing a high endothelial venule. Note the lymphocyte that appears to be passing between endothelial cells.

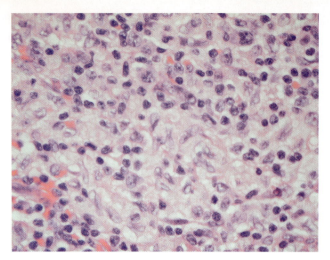

FIGURE 2.12 Section of paracortex showing many inter-digitating reticulum cells. The twisted grooved nuclei of these cells have an appearance said to resemble a 'wrung-out dishcloth'. They have abundant, ill-defined, pale pink cytoplasm.

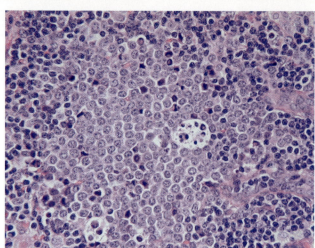

FIGURE 2.15 High-power view of an island of plasmacy-toid monocytes. Note the regular rounded nuclei of these cells and their amphophilic cytoplasm. Many apoptotic cells are present together with two 'tingible body' macrophages.

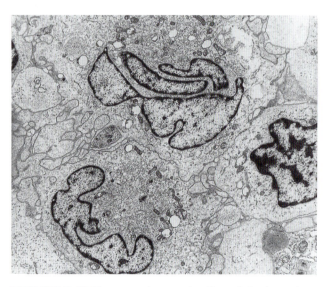

FIGURE 2.13 Electron micrograph of interdigitating reticu-lum cells. Note the complexity of the nuclear shape and the interdigitating cell membranes that give this cell its name.

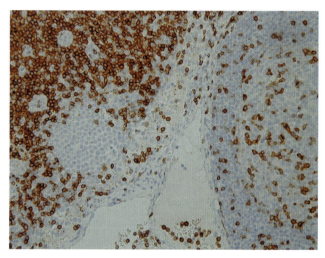

FIGURE 2.16 Section of reactive lymph node stained for CD3. Note scattered T-cells in the reactive follicle (right) and more closely packed T-cells in the paracortex (left). The island of plasmacytoid monocytes is unstained.

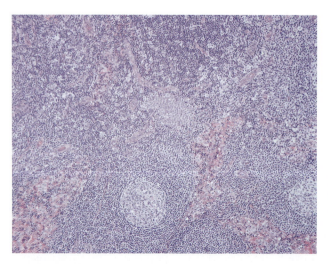

FIGURE 2.14 Section of reactive lymph node showing two follicles and an island of plasmacytoid monocytes.

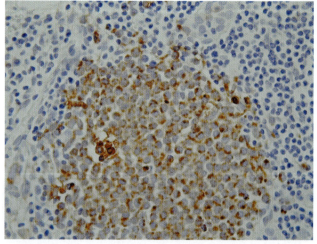

FIGURE 2.17 Island of plasmacytoid monocytes stained for CD68. Note strong granular staining of the plasmacytoid monocytes and strong staining of a 'tingible body' macrophage.

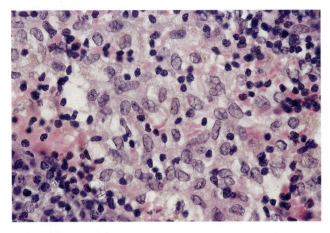

FIGURE 2.18 Sinus lining cells showing oval or bean-shaped nuclei with inconspicuous nucleoli and abundant pale-staining cytoplasm.

uniform size with rounded, often eccentric, nuclei that lack the characteristic clumped chromatin of plasma cells. In Giemsa-stained preparations the cytoplasm is basophilic and electron microscopy shows stacks of rough endoplasmic reticulum. Apoptotic cells are characteristically seen within clusters of plasmacytoid monocytes, although the proliferative activity of these cells is low. Their accumulation and survival is cytokine dependent and they are thought to be precursors of antigen-presenting dendritic cells.

MEDULLARY CORDS

Medullary cords occur towards the hilum of the lymph node and contain a variable mixture of small lymphocytes, blast cells and plasma cells. Plasma cells are particularly prominent in chronic inflammatory diseases, such as rheumatoid disease.

SINUSES

Afferent lymphatics enter the lymph node along its convex surface and an efferent vessel leaves from the concave hilum of the node. Lymph enters the subcapsular sinus and then percolates through the network of medullary sinuses. The sinuses are defined by a scaffolding of type IV collagen to which are attached the sinus lining cells. These cells have dendritic processes and attach to each other through desmosomes. They are not phagocytic and appear to act as antigen presenting cells. In addition to the sinus lining cells, the sinuses contain variable numbers of mononuclear cells, including phagocytic histiocytes.

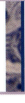

3 REACTIVE AND INFECTIVE LYMPHADENOPATHY

We have categorized this disparate group of lymph-adenopathies on the basis of their most prominent histological feature (Box 3.1). This is to some extent arbitrary, since some have overlapping features and these may vary at different stages of the disease. Biopsy is most likely to be performed in patients with persistent lymph-adenopathy, often to exclude malignancy. Well-taken, well-fixed, whole lymph node biopsies are desirable in such cases because a number of reactive lymph-adenopathies may closely mimic malignant lymphoma.

FOLLICULAR HYPERPLASIA

NON-SPECIFIC FOLLICULAR HYPERPLASIA

Follicular hyperplasia is probably the most common pattern of lymph node reaction seen and is character-ized by enlarged follicles with prominent germinal centres. It is often accompanied by the presence of plasma cells in the medullary cords and throughout the interfollicular parenchyma. The causes of reactive

---

BOX 3.1: Patterns of reactive and infective hyperplasia

FOLLICULAR HYPERPLASIA
Non-specific follicular
    hyperplasia
Rheumatoid lymphadenopathy
Syphilis
Toxoplasmosis
Kimura disease
Measles
Human immunodeficiency virus (HIV)
    lymphadenitis
Progressive transformation of germinal centres
Castleman disease

PARACORTICAL EXPANSION
Dermatopathic lymphadenopathy
Kikuchi–Fujimoto disease
Systemic lupus erythematosus
Viral lymphadenitis, including infectious
    mononucleosis
Drug-induced lymphadenopathy

SINUS EXPANSION
Rosai–Dorfman disease (sinus histiocytosis
    with massive lymphadenopathy)
Langerhans cell histiocytosis
Lipogranulomatous reaction
Silicone lymphadenopathy and storage diseases

**GRANULOMATOUS
LYMPHADENOPATHY**
Suppurative: Cat scratch, lymphogranuloma
    venereum, tularaemia, *Yersinia*, *Listeria*,
    Corynebacterium

Epithelioid Granulomas
Necrotizing: Tuberculosis, atypical mycobacteria,
    leprosy, fungi
Non-necrotizing: Sarcoidosis, berylliosis,
    protozoa and metazoa, lymph nodes draining
    carcinoma
Reaction to foreign materials

follicular hyperplasia generally include antigen challenges that stimulate a B-cell response. Ancillary diagnostic procedures identify many of the aetiologic agents but in the absence of demonstrable infecting micro-organisms and any specific histologic feature that may point to the aetiology, this reaction is termed 'non-specific hyperplasia'. Such non-specific reactions are more common in children and young adults, and are often seen in nodes draining infected sites, such as tonsils, skin or intestinal tract. In reactive lymphadenopathy, the follicles retain a distinct mantle of small lymphocytes, and the germinal centres may show polarization of the centroblasts and centrocytes. They are generally distributed predominantly in the cortex of the node and are often irregular in shape and size. Reactive germinal centres show a large number of mitotic figures and numerous apoptotic bodies that are frequently phagocytosed by 'tingible body macrophages'.

RHEUMATOID LYMPHADENOPATHY

The lymphadenopathy in rheumatoid arthritis is not limited to nodes draining affected joints but may often be generalized as part of this systemic disease. There is marked follicular hyperplasia. The enlarged germinal centres may contain amorphous periodic acid–Schiff (PAS)-positive hyaline deposits and infrequently sarcoid-like granulomas may accompany the follicular hyperplasia. Large numbers of plasma cells, often with Russell bodies, infiltrate the medullary cords and may also be present within germinal centres.

Gold lymphadenopathy is a complication of long-standing intramuscular injections of colloidal gold for rheumatoid arthritis. The lymph nodes show changes similar to those of rheumatoid lymphadenopathy. In addition, there is sinus histiocytosis with histiocytes and giant cells containing black pigment. This pigment gives a characteristic orange–red birefringence in polarized light.

SYPHILIS

In primary syphilis, the site of entry of *Treponema pallidum* is characterized by a chancre that heals after 2–4 weeks but the treponemes spread from the chancre to regional lymph nodes, which become enlarged, hard and painless. Secondary syphilis begins 6–8 weeks after infection, and is manifested by generalized lymphadenopathy with localized or generalized skin and mucosal eruptions. After a latency of as long as 2 years with occasional relapses, tertiary syphilis develops with the formation of gummata, ulcers and nodules in various organs, including the cardiovascular and central nervous systems. The lymphadenopathy that accompanies all three stages of the disease is due to persistence of the organisms with continuous antigenic stimulation of B- and T-cells. The former is represented by marked follicular hyperplasia that extends into the medulla. This is accompanied by expansion of the paracortex and marked fibrosis of the capsule, the fibrosis sometimes penetrating into the node. Plasmacytosis is prominent within the medullary cords. Small non-caseating epithelioid granulomas are sometimes present with single so-called naked giant cells in the paracortex. There is arteritis and phlebitis of the numerous vessels that form in the capsule and pericapsular tissues, and these are characterized by a prominent cuff of plasma cells and lymphocytes.

Silver stains reveal the spirochaetes in the walls of high-endothelial venules and capsular vessels in all three stages of the disease.

TOXOPLASMA LYMPHADENOPATHY

Lymphadenitis is the most frequent manifestation of symptomatic toxoplasmosis. *Toxoplasma gondii*, a coccidian parasite, is one of the most prevalent and geographically widespread protozoan infections of man. The histological changes of toxoplasmic lymphadenitis are a mixed pattern of prominent follicular hyperplasia and monocytoid B-cell hyperplasia with small to large clusters of epithelioid cells in the paracortex and sometimes extending into the germinal centres. Very rarely, parasitic cysts are found, usually within the cortical sinus of the node. These cysts do not appear to evoke a tissue response and the low rate of detection of *Toxoplasma* genomes by polymerase chain reaction has raised the suspicion that the lymphadenitis may be a reaction to protozoan antigens rather that to direct contact with the organisms.

KIMURA DISEASE

Kimura disease is a self-limiting condition that is prevalent among but not exclusive to Orientals, with a striking male predominance. If untreated, this idiopathic condition usually remains static and may show regression. The nodes involved measure up to a few centimetres in diameter and multiple enlarged nodes may become matted. The histological changes are characterized by follicular hyperplasia, paracortical expansion with prominent high endothelial venules and marked eosinophilic infiltration. There is often a proteinaceous precipitate in the germinal centres and immunostains reveal immunoglobulin E (IgE) deposited on the follicular dendritic network. The germinal centres may show foci of necrosis or folliculolysis. There is an accompanying eosinophilic infiltration of the germinal centres that can form eosinophilic microabscesses. Eosinophils infiltrate the sinuses and paracortex where microabscesses may also form. The expanded paracortex contains plasma cells, small lymphocytes, mast cells and occasional Warthin–Finkeldey type giant cells. Patchy fibrosis may occur around venules.

HUMAN IMMUNODEFICIENCY VIRUS/ACQUIRED IMMUNE DEFICIENCY SYNDROME (HIV/AIDS) LYMPHADENITIS

Persistent generalized lymphadenopathy accompanied by weight loss, fever, night sweats, malaise, diarrhoea and hypergammaglobulinaemia may be a presenting manifestation of HIV/AIDS.

Human immunodeficiency virus shows strong tropism for lymphoid tissues, especially CD4-positive T-cells, monocytes and dendritic cells. In the acute phase of the infection, HIV infects mononuclear cells in the peripheral blood, which migrate to lymphoid organs causing acute reactive lymphadenitis. Macrophages and dendritic cells in lymph nodes form the reservoirs for the virus while circulating T-cells disseminate the virus. The result of continued infection causes cytopathic destruction of CD4+ T-cells and dendritic cells in germinal centres so that the latter involute. Opportunistic infections may supervene.

Lymph node histology progresses with evolution of the disease through the following stages:

* florid follicular hyperplasia;
* mixed follicular hyperplasia and follicular involution;
* follicular involution;
* lymphocyte depletion.

Lymph nodes at the stage of florid follicular hyperplasia show very prominent, often irregular (geographic) follicles. The mantle cells are often attenuated and in places may be disrupted. Naked germinal centres may be seen. There is often marginal zone B-cell hyperplasia. Multinucleated giant cells of the Warthin–Finkeldey type are scattered randomly in the parenchyma.

Follicular lysis follows infiltration of the germinal centres by small lymphocytes resulting in disruption of the follicles. PAS-positive material accumulates in the follicles making them less cellular. Follicular lysis is accompanied by progressive plasma cell accumulation.

Lymphocyte depletion represents the burnt-out stage of HIV/AIDS lymphadenitis with atrophic follicles, lymphocyte depletion and extensive, diffuse vascular proliferation. The follicles are small and depleted of lymphoid cells and contain thick collagen-ensheathed vessels surrounded by deposits of PAS-positive material. The follicular atrophy may progress to complete hyalinization, and interfollicular and paracortical zones show lymphocyte depletion and extensive vascularization. There is a prominence of plasma cells and diffuse fibrosis so that the overall appearance is that of an exhausted, burnt-out node.

The presence of HIV in infected nodes can be demonstrated with immunostaining to various HIV antigens, such as the core protein p24. Staining for this antigen is localized to the follicular dendritic cells similar to the distribution of the virus detected by electron microscopy. HIV RNA can also be demonstrated by *in-situ* hybridization and the polymerase chain reaction.

PROGRESSIVE TRANSFORMATION OF GERMINAL CENTRES

Progressive transformation of germinal centres (PTGC) is most commonly seen in adolescent and young adult males, presenting as solitary painless lymphadenopathy, sometimes of long duration. The cervical nodes are most commonly involved, axillary and inguinal nodes much less frequently. The disease runs a benign course but it may be recurrent. Rare cases show a synchronous or metachronous association with nodular lymphocyte-predominant Hodgkin lymphoma (NLPHL).

Lymph nodes are usually considerably enlarged and may have been present for many months. They show one or several expanded follicles interspersed between the reactive follicles. The expansion of the follicles and disruption of the germinal centres is caused by the influx of mantle cells. This is seen most clearly with immunohistochemistry. Mantle cells stain strongly with antibodies to immunoglobulin D (IgD) and CD79a, and can be seen breaking up the germinal centres into small clusters of cells. Antibodies to follicular dendritic cells (CD21, CD23, CD35) show an expanded dendritic cell network. Loose clusters of epithelioid histiocytes may be seen in PTGC; in some cases these surround the expanded follicle.

The main differential diagnosis of PTGC is with NLPHL. In the former, the expanded follicles are scattered amongst reactive follicles; in the latter, any residual reactive follicles are compressed towards the periphery of the node. Unlike the individual L and H cells (popcorn cells) seen within nodules of NLPHL, the cells at the centre of the nodules of PTGC consist of clusters of centroblasts.

CASTLEMAN DISEASE

Castleman disease is conveniently divided into three categories:

- hyaline vascular;
- plasma cell variant – localized;
- multicentric Castleman disease.

There may appear to be some overlap between these categories, possibly owing to the fact that the follicles in the plasma cell variant become more hyaline with time.

HYALINE VASCULAR CASTLEMAN DISEASE

Hyaline vascular Castleman disease (HVCD) occurs most commonly in young adults and presents most frequently in the mediastinum. Peripheral lymph nodes may be involved, as also may be various extranodal sites. The lesion is usually solitary and not accompanied by systemic symptoms.

Histologically, HVCD shows characteristic follicles with a broad mantle of small lymphocytes that often assume a concentric onion-skin pattern. The centres of the follicles are hypocellular, consisting mainly of endothelial cells and dendritic reticulum cells, some of which may show nuclear atypia. Occasional follicles, depending on the plane of section, show penetration through the mantle by vessels ensheathed with collagen giving a lollipop appearance.

The interfollicular tissues are composed predominantly of a network of vessels on a thick collagenous scaffold, a feature well demonstrated in sections stained for reticulin. Scattered or clustered small lymphocytes, plasma cells and plasmacytoid monocytes are seen amongst these vessels. Sinus structures are not usually identifiable.

Typical HVCD is so characteristic that it is easily recognizable. Difficulties may arise when few or many hyaline vascular follicles are found in what otherwise appears to be a reactive lymph node, such as might be seen in the late stages of HIV infection. These cases, in contrast with HVCD, usually show some residual sinus structure, contain more plasma cells and lack an interfollicular vascular network.

Hyaline vascular Castleman disease is a benign proliferation that is usually cured by local resection. It has a rare association with dendritic cell sarcoma.

CASTLEMAN DISEASE PLASMA CELL VARIANT – LOCALIZED

Castleman disease plasma cell variant – localized (PCD) has a wide age spectrum. It presents most commonly with abdominal lymphadenopathy, involving one or a group of nodes. Mediastinal and peripheral lymphadenopathy are much less common than in HVCD. Patients typically have systemic symptoms and abnormal laboratory tests: anaemia, raised polyclonal gamma globulin, elevated erythrocyte sedimentation rate (ESR) and increased plasma cells in bone marrow. These symptoms disappear and the laboratory tests revert to normal following surgical removal of the affected nodes. The systemic effects appear to be mediated by interleukin-6 (IL-6) secreted by the affected nodes.

Histologically, PCD shows follicular hyperplasia with a narrow mantle zone surrounded by sheets of mature plasma cells. The density of the plasma cells often obscures the underlying sinus structure, although this is usually identifiable in areas. In the majority of cases of PCD the plasma cells show polytypic immunoglobulin light chain expression, over one-third show light-chain restriction (usually lambda light chain).

The main histological differential diagnosis of PCD is with reactive lymphadenopathies showing marked plasmacytosis, as seen in rheumatoid disease and syphilis. In these nodes, the underlying sinus structure is usually more apparent and the interfollicular infiltrate less uniformly plasmacytic.

MULTICENTRIC CASTLEMAN DISEASE

Multicentric Castleman disease (MCD) occurs in an older age group than PCD or HVCD. It may appear as a primary disease or in association with HIV infection, Kaposi sarcoma, plasma cell neoplasms, malignant lymphomas and autoimmune disease. In common with PCD it is associated with systemic symptoms and abnormal laboratory findings. The underlying pathogenesis appears to be the overproduction of IL-6 either from endogenous sources or from the viral homologue of IL-6 produced by human herpes virus 8 (HHV-8). It has been suggested that MCD should be called IL-6 lymphadenopathy.

The histopathology of MCD is similar to that of PCD. It may progress to a burnt-out phase with abundant hyaline vascular germinal centres, when it might be interpreted as HVCD or mixed HVCD/PCD.

The POEMS syndrome is associated with MCD in approximately 60 per cent of cases. The features of this syndrome (polyneuropathy, organomegaly, endocrine abnormalities, monoclonal gammopathy, skin rashes) are thought to result from the production of autoantibodies and to cytokine abnormalities.

Patients with MCD have a poor prognosis.

BOX 3.2: Rheumatoid lymphadenopathy

- Lymphadenopathy may be widespread
- Follicular hyperplasia
- Follicles may contain plasma cells
- Mantle zone retained
- Plasma cell infiltration of medullary cords

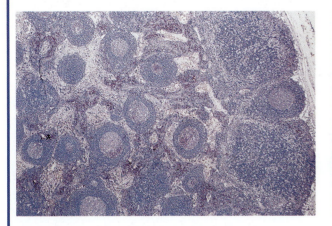

FIGURE 3.1 Rheumatoid lymphadenopathy: lymph node stained with methyl-green pyronin. The node shows follicular hyperplasia with numerous red (pyroninophilic) plasma cells in the medullary cords.

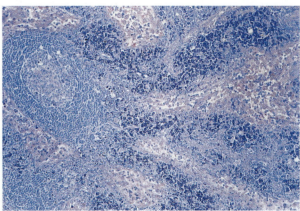

FIGURE 3.2 Rheumatoid lymphadenopathy: lymph node stained by Giemsa stain. The deep basophilia of the plasma cell cytoplasm highlights these cells in the medullary cords.

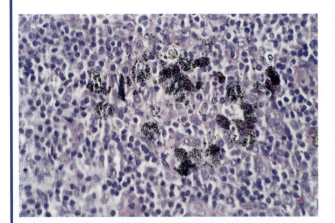

FIGURE 3.3 'Gold lymphadenopathy'. Axillary lymph node from a patient with rheumatoid disease treated with colloidal gold. Black pigment is seen within histiocytes.

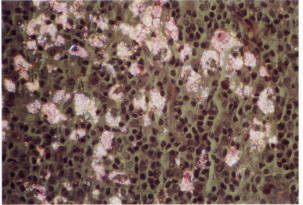

FIGURE 3.4 'Gold lymphadenopathy' viewed in polarized light showing characteristic orange–red birefringence.

BOX 3.3: Syphilitic lymphadenopathy

- Generalized lymphadenopathy a feature of secondary syphilis
- Follicular hyperplasia
- Plasma cells expand medullary cords
- Epithelial cell clusters in paracortex

- Naked giant cells
- Capsular fibrosis
- Arteritis and phlebitis of capsular vessels
- Perivascular lymphoplasmacytic cuffing
- Spirochaetes demonstrated by silver stains

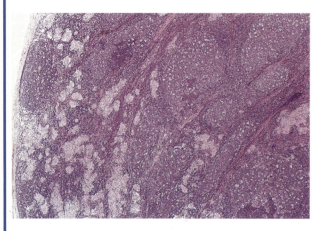

FIGURE 3.5 Secondary syphilis. Lymph node showing marked follicular hyperplasia with small epithelioid granulomas in the paracortex.

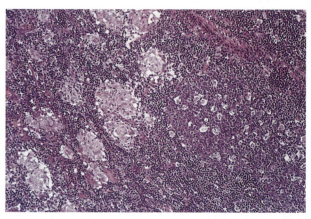

FIGURE 3.6 Secondary syphilis. Lymph node showing epithelioid cell clusters in the paracortex adjacent to a reactive follicle.

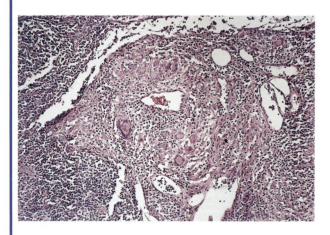

FIGURE 3.7 Syphilitic lymph node showing marked venulitis with giant cells.

BOX 3.4: Toxoplasmic lymphadenitis

- Prominent follicular hyperplasia
- Monocytoid B-cell hyperplasia
- Epithelioid cell clusters that often impinge on germinal centres

- Toxoplasma pseudocysts filled with merozoites are exceptional

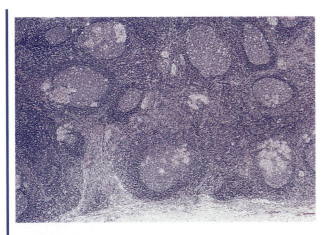

FIGURE 3.8 Toxoplasmosis. Lymph node showing marked follicular hyperplasia and numerous small epithelioid cell clusters.

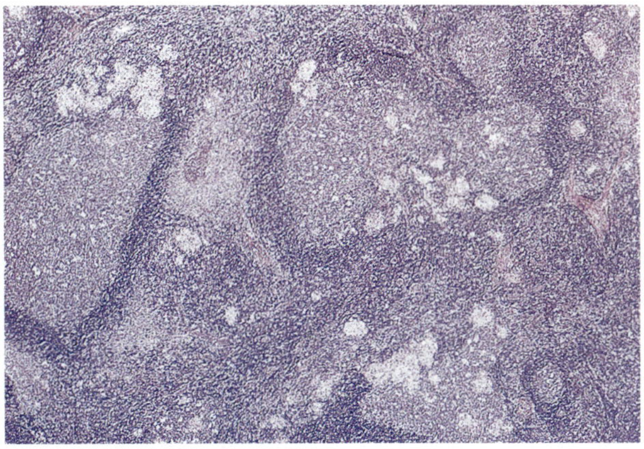

FIGURE 3.9 Toxoplasmosis. The epithelioid cell clusters appear to encroach on and enter the germinal centres. A collection of monocytoid B-cells is seen between the two germinal centres.

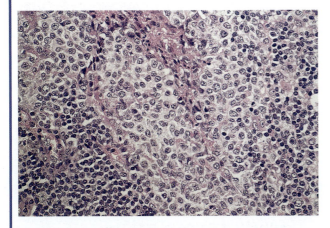

FIGURE 3.10 Toxoplasmosis. Prominent monocytoid B-cells distributed in and around a sinus.

BOX 3.5: Kimura disease

- Common in Asians, male predominance
- Enlarged lymph nodes in neck and peri-auricular region, may be matted
- Occasional involvement of salivary glands
- Blood eosinophilia
- Florid follicular and germinal centre hyper-plasia with proteinaceous precipitate

- IgE deposition on follicular dendritic cells
- Paracortical expansion by plasma cells, small lymphocytes and mast cells
- Marked eosinophil infiltration of germinal centres, paracortex and medulla with microabscess formation
- Warthin–Finkeldey-type polykaryocytes

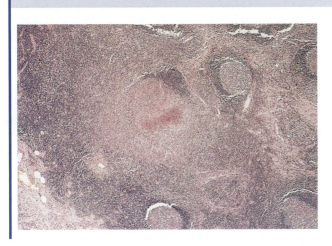

FIGURE 3.11 Kimura disease. Lymph node shows follicular hyperplasia. One follicle shows necrosis and an eosinophil micro abscess.

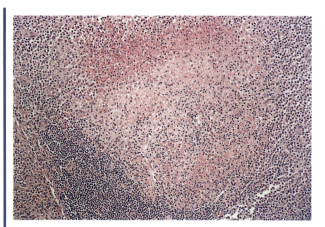

FIGURE 3.12 Kimura disease. High-power view of the follicle containing an eosinophil microabscess.

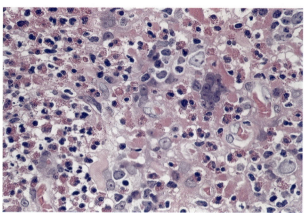

FIGURE 3.13 Kimura disease. Follicle centre largely replaced by eosinophils and amorphous eosinophilic material. Also shown is a follicular dendritic cell polykaryon.

BOX 3.6: Human immunodeficiency virus lymphadenitis

APPROPRIATE CLINICAL SETTING
- Fever, weight loss, diarrhoea, hypergammaglobulinaemia
- Persons at risk for infection
- Palpable lymph nodes at two or more sites
- Decreased peripheral CD4+ T-cells
- Reversed CD4+ /CD8+ T-cell ratio
- Positive human immunodeficiency virus (HIV) antigen or antibody test

FLORID FOLLICULAR HYPERPLASIA (ACUTE STAGE)
- Hyperplastic, irregular follicles
- Mantle may be attenuated or disrupted
- Monocytoid B-cell hyperplasia
- Warthin–Finkeldey giant cells

FOLLICULAR INVOLUTION (SUBACUTE/CHRONIC STAGE)
- Follicular effacement
- Germinal centre involution with accumulation of hyaline material
- Lymphocyte depletion in paracortex
- Plasma cell accumulation in paracortex
- Vascular proliferation in paracortex

LYMPHOCYTE DEPLETION (BURNOUT)
- Atrophic or absent follicles
- Hyalinized germinal centres with prominent thick vessels and periodic acid–Schiff (PAS)-positive deposits
- Lymphocyte depletion in paracortex
- Extensive vascular proliferation and fibrosis

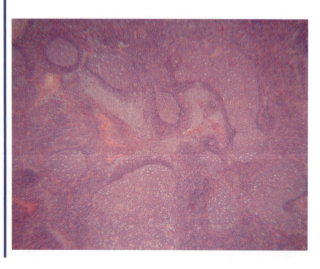

FIGURE 3.14 Human immunodeficiency virus lymphadenopathy. Lymph node showing follicular hyperplasia with large irregular germinal centres. Islands of pale-staining monocytoid B-cells can be seen in the centre of the field.

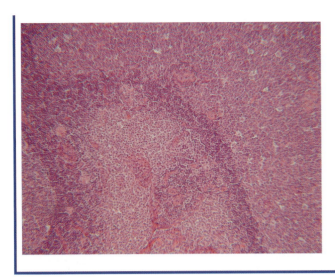

FIGURE 3.15 Human immunodeficiency virus lymphadenopathy. High-power view showing part of a germinal centre and an island of monocytoid B-cells.

BOX 3.7: Progressive transformation of germinal centres

- Most common in young males
- May be recurrent
- Single, asymptomatic, enlarged node
- Expanded follicles in a background of follicular hyperplasia

- Thick mantle around expanded follicles
- Mantle cells infiltrate germinal centres, which break up into small groups of centroblasts

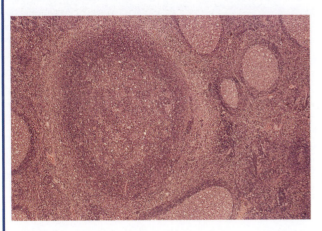

FIGURE 3.16 Progressive transformation of germinal centres. Section showing a 'transformed' expanded germinal centre with adjacent reactive lymphoid follicles.

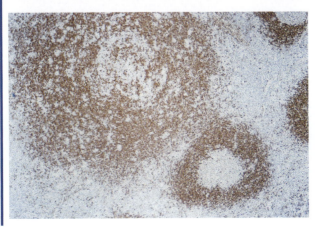

FIGURE 3.17 Progressive transformation of germinal centres. Section stained for CD79a showing strong positive staining of mantle cells. The 'transformed' follicle is expanded and broken up by mantle cells. Staining for immunoglobulin D would show a similar appearance.

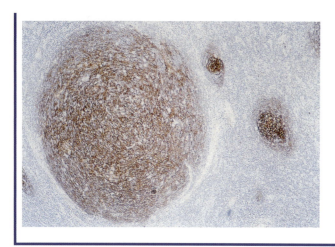

FIGURE 3.18 Progressive transformation of germinal centres. Section stained for CD21 showing follicular dendritic cells. The 'transformed' follicle shows an expanded network of follicular dendritic cells in comparison with the tight networks seen in the adjacent reactive follicles.

BOX 3.8: Castleman disease

HYALINE VASCULAR CASTLEMAN DISEASE

- Most common in young adults
- Commonly presents in mediastinum
- Hyaline follicles consist mainly of endothelial cells and dendritic reticulum cells
- Mantle zone shows onion-skin layering
- Interfollicular areas vascular
- Sinus structure not usually visible

CASTLEMAN DISEASE PLASMA CELL VARIANT – LOCALIZED

- Wide age range
- Systemic symptoms
- Anaemia, hyperglobulinaemia, elevated erythrocyte sedimentation rate (ESR), increased plasma cells in bone marrow
- Abdominal nodes most commonly involved
- Follicular hyperplasia with narrow mantle zones

- Dense interfollicular infiltrate of plasma cells obscures underlying architecture
- One-third of cases show light-chain restriction

MULTICENTRIC CASTLEMAN DISEASE

- Older age groups
- May be primary or associated with other diseases such as HIV/acquired immune deficiency syndrome (AIDS)
- Overproduction of interleukin-6 from endogenous sources or from human herpes virus (HHV)-6
- Histology similar to localized disease
- 60 per cent of cases associated with POEMS syndrome (polyneuropathy, organomegaly, endocrine abnormalities, monoclonal gammopathy, skin rashes)

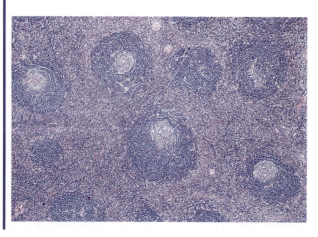

FIGURE 3.19 Castleman disease, hyaline vascular type. Note hyalinized follicles and lack of sinus structures.

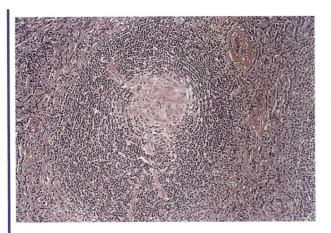

FIGURE 3.20 Castleman disease, hyaline vascular type. Follicle showing hyalinization of the germinal centre with penetrating vessels, onion-skin layering of the mantle cells and vascularized interfollicular tissue.

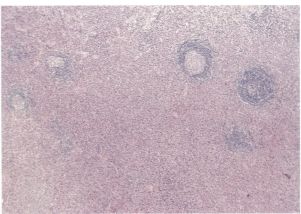

FIGURE 3.21 Castleman disease, plasma cell variant. Reactive follicles in a background of plasma cells. No sinus structure visible.

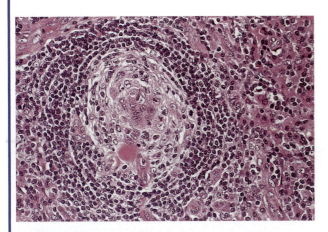

FIGURE 3.22 Castleman disease, plasma cell variant. Hyalinized follicle composed mainly of dendritic and endothelial cells surrounded by plasma cells.

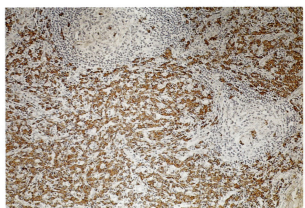

FIGURE 3.23 Castleman disease, plasma cell variant. Immunohistochemistry shows monotypic lambda light-chain staining.

PARACORTICAL EXPANSION

VIRAL LYMPHADENOPATHY

In using lymph node architecture to categorize reactive and infective lymphadenopathies, the viral lymphadenopathies present the problem that they may be associated with both follicular and paracortical expansion. We have therefore divided them on the basis of their most prominent feature, including HIV/AIDS under 'follicular hyperplasia' and infectious mononucleosis and other viral lymphadenopathies under 'paracortical expansion'.

MEASLES LYMPHADENOPATHY

The measles virus, a paramyxovirus, produces a marked systemic lymphoid response as the virus multiplies in macrophages and lymphocytes in the unimmunized patient. Following vaccination with live attenuated virus, there may be associated lymphadenitis. The infection is characterized by a marked proliferation of immunoblasts in the paracortex accompanied by follicular hyperplasia. Nodal architecture may be partially obliterated by diffuse sheets of immunoblasts with a relative depletion of lymphocytes so that a mottled appearance is produced. Scattered among these cells and within follicles are Warthin–Finkeldey cells, which also appear in various hyperplastic lymphoid tissues during the prodromal stage of the infection. These large syncytial polykaryocytes are 25–150 μm in diameter with as many as 50 nuclei; they result from the fusion of various cell types mediated by the measles virus.

INFECTIOUS MONONUCLEOSIS LYMPHADENOPATHY

The Epstein–Barr virus (EBV) infects susceptible lymphoid cells in the oropharynx and persists as a latent virus throughout life. Infection in infants is usually symptomless or trivial. When older patients are infected, the disease may be severe and may simulate lymphoma. In the acute infection, the virus replicates in perifollicular B-cells, stimulating a vigorous humoral and cellular immune response.

Involved lymph nodes are enlarged but not matted. They may show varying degrees of follicular hyperplasia but the most striking feature is paracortical expansion. Large numbers of blast cells, many of immunoblast morphology, are seen within the paracortex. Immunohistochemistry shows that these are of both B- and T-cell phenotype. Occasionally, atypical cells and cells resembling Hodgkin/Reed–Sternberg cells are seen. However, this is a feature more frequently encountered in tonsils than in lymph nodes.

OTHER VIRAL LYMPHADENOPATHIES

Other common viruses that cause lymphadenitis include cytomegalovirus, Herpes simplex, varicella–Herpes zoster and vaccinia; however, such cases are rarely biopsied. Although there may be some element of follicular hyperplasia, such nodes usually show a predominant pattern of paracortical hyperplasia. Monocytoid B-cell hyperplasia may be seen at some stages of the infection and areas of necrosis may occur. Characteristic intranuclear and/or cytoplasmic inclusions may be seen. Immunostaining with specific antibodies is available for cytomegalovirus, Herpes simplex and Herpes zoster.

DERMATOPATHIC LYMPHADENOPATHY

Dermatopathic lymphadenopathy (DL) shows paracortical hyperplasia resulting from the accumulation of interdigitating reticulum cells (IDRC), Langerhans cells (LC), histiocytes containing lipid and melanin, and paracortical T-cells. DL represents the reaction of a superficial lymph node to the drainage of skin antigens and melanin from various chronic dermatoses. In

patients with cerebriform cutaneous T-cell lymphomas (mycosis fungoides and Sézary syndrome), it may be difficult or impossible to determine whether lymph nodes showing DL contain neoplastic T-cells. In such cases, it is necessary to look for T-cell receptor clonality in order to confirm neoplastic infiltration.

Grossly, the enlarged lymph node may show a distinct rim of pigment immediately beneath the capsule. The nodal architecture is preserved and there is marked paracortical expansion comprising irregular pale staining nodules of IDRC and LC, histiocytes and intermingled T-cells. Scattered phagocytic histiocytes are found intermingled with the IDRC. These may have foamy cytoplasm and contain ingested melanin and lipid. IDRC and LC express S100 protein, which provides a good immunohistochemical marker for DL.

KIKUCHI DISEASE

Kikuchi disease (synonyms: Kikuchi–Fujimoto disease, histiocytic necrotizing lymphadenitis) is a self-limiting disease occurring predominantly in adolescent and young adult females. It is more prevalent in Asia than in the rest of the world. The most common presentation is with one or more enlarged cervical lymph nodes that are frequently painful and may be associated with fever and systemic symptoms. Other superficial lymph nodes are much less frequently affected. The aetiology is unknown.

The histology of Kikuchi disease varies as the disease progresses. In the early stages, there is variable follicular hyperplasia with expansion of the paracortex by small lymphocytes, B- and T-cell blasts, plasmacytoid monocytes and histiocytes. Apoptosis is usually prominent among these cells. As the disease progresses, areas of necrosis appear. Neutrophils are not associated with these areas of necrosis, presumably because the cells are undergoing apoptosis. As the apoptosis and necrosis progresses, the number of histiocytes increases until they become the predominant cell type. Many of these histiocytes contain ingested cell debris and characteristically have crescentic nuclei.

Immunohistochemical markers for CD68 will identify histiocytes and plasmacytoid monocytes. Both B- and T-cell antibodies will often identify B- and T-cell blasts among the non-necrotic cells. The majority of the small lymphocytes are CD8 positive T-cells.

Kikuchi disease must be differentiated from non-Hodgkin lymphoma. In the proliferative phase of the disease the appearance of sheets of blast cells, as also is the case in infectious mononucleosis, may appear alarming. The presence of an underlying normal nodal structure, and the morphological and immunohistochemical heterogeneity of the cells distinguishes Kikuchi disease from lymphoma. Kikuchi disease may be confused with other diseases that cause lymph node necrosis in which fragmented neutrophil nuclei may give an appearance suggesting preceding apoptosis. Markers for granulocytes, such as CD15, will identify these neutrophils, cells that are almost invariably absent from Kikuchi disease.

SYSTEMIC LUPUS ERYTHEMATOSUS LYMPHADENOPATHY

Lymphadenopathy may occur in patients with systemic lupus erythematosus (SLE), but in practice biopsy of such nodes is rare, probably because other manifestations of the disease have already established the diagnosis. The histological findings in lymph nodes from patients with SLE have features in common with Kikuchi disease and it is probably wise to bring this to the attention of the clinicians when reporting Kikuchi disease. Features that differentiate the two conditions are the presence of haematoxylin bodies (aggregates of DNA and anti-DNA antibodies), vasculitis, DNA deposition on blood vessels and plasma cell infiltrates in SLE.

DRUG-INDUCED LYMPHADENOPATHY

Drug-induced lymphadenopathy is most commonly seen in patients exhibiting hypersensitivity to anticonvulsant drugs (carbamazepine, dilantin, phenytoin) but it may also be seen in association with hypersensitivity to other drugs. Patients typically show fever, skin rashes and generalized lymphadenopathy with eosinophilia.

Lymph nodes show a predominantly paracortical expansion with a population of B- and T-cell blasts, small lymphocytes, histiocytes, neutrophils and eosinophils. The blast cells may have prominent nucleoli but they do not exhibit atypia.

BOX 3.9: Measles lymphadenitis

- Measles infection or recent vaccination
- Nodal and extranodal lymphoid tissue involved
- Follicular hyperplasia and paracortical expansion
- Mottled appearance due to marked proliferation of immunoblasts and relative depletion of lymphocytes in the paracortex
- Warthin–Finkeldey giant cells

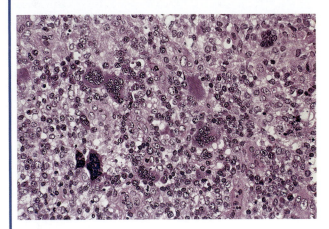

FIGURE 3.24 Measles lymphadenopathy. Warthin–Finkeldey giant cells in paracortex of lymph node following measles vaccination.

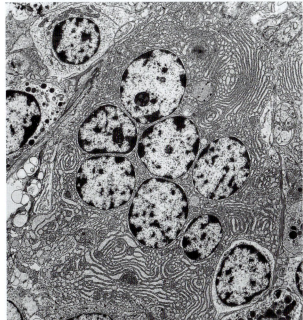

FIGURE 3.25 Electron micrograph of Warthin–Finkeldey giant cell formed by the fusion of plasma cells in a case of measles lymphadenopathy.

BOX 3.10: Infectious mononucleosis lymphadenitis

- Teenagers and young adults affected
- Paracortical expansion
- Numerous B- and T-immunoblasts present in paracortex

- Atypical Hodgkin/Reed–Sternberg-like cells may be seen, but are more common in the tonsil than in lymph nodes

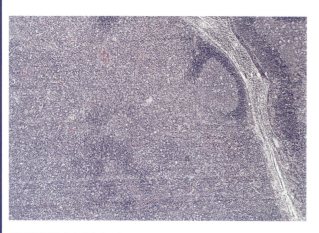

FIGURE 3.26 Infectious mononucleosis lymphadenopathy. Low-power view showing paracortical blast cell hyperplasia partially surrounding a reactive follicle.

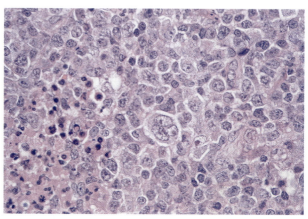

FIGURE 3.27 Infectious mononucleosis lymphadenopathy. Paracortex showing blastic hyperplasia; note multinucleated cell and apoptotic nuclei.

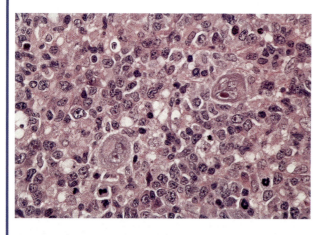

FIGURE 3.28 Infectious mononucleosis lymphadenopathy showing cells resembling Reed–Sternberg cells in the paracortex.

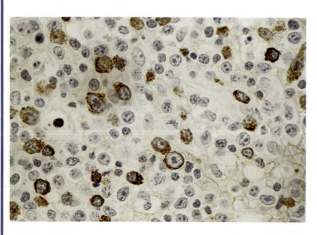

FIGURE 3.29 Infectious mononucleosis lymphadenopathy. Immunoperoxidase technique showing immunoglobulin M positive B-cell blasts in the paracortex.

BOX 3.11: Dermatopathic lymphadenopathy

- Superficial lymph nodes draining chronic dermatoses
- Cut surface of node may show subcapsular rim of pigment

- Paracortical expansion with aggregates of interdigitating reticulum cells and Langerhans cells
- Scattered macrophages containing lipid and melanin

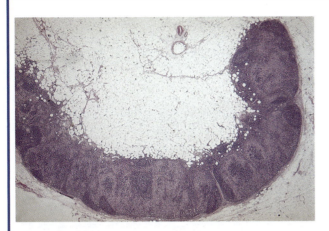

FIGURE 3.30 Dermatopathic lymphadenopathy. Axillary lymph node showing expanded pale-staining paracortex.

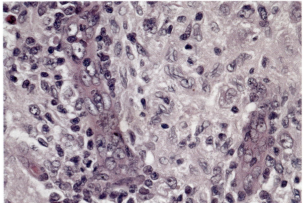

FIGURE 3.31 Dermatopathic lymphadenopathy. High-power view showing characteristic interdigitating reticulum cells with elongated grooved and twisted nuclei and abundant pale cytoplasm.

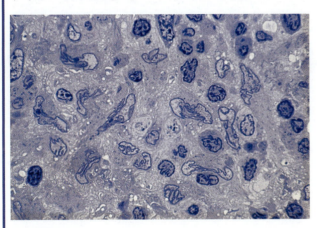

FIGURE 3.32 Dermatopathic lymphadenopathy. Plastic-embedded section showing the characteristic morphology of interdigitating reticulum cells.

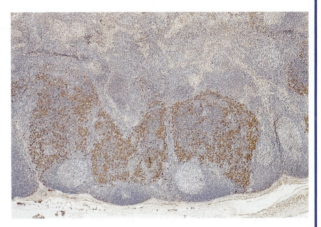

FIGURE 3.33 Dermatopathic lymphadenopathy. Section stained for S100 protein showing the expanded network of interdigitating reticulum cells in the paracortex.

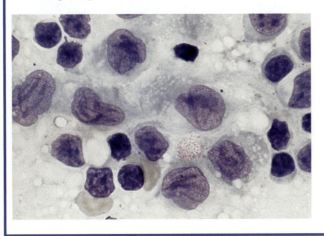

FIGURE 3.34 Dermatopathic lymphadenopathy, imprint cytology. The interdigitating reticulum cells have grooved nuclei and abundant pale-staining cytoplasm.

BOX 3.12: Kikuchi disease

- Most common in Asia
- Most common in adolescent and young adult females
- Cervical lymphadenopathy, often painful Other nodes less commonly affected
- Systemic symptoms and fever common
- Paracortical expansion with small lymphocytes, blast cells, plasmacytoid monocytes and histiocytes

- Plasma cells uncommon
- Widespread apoptosis and areas of necrosis without neutrophils
- Phagocytic histiocytes characteristically have crescentic nuclei

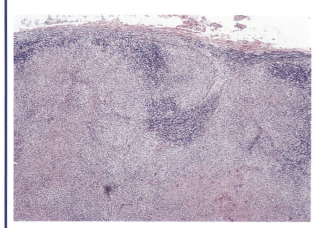

FIGURE 3.35 Kikuchi disease. Lymph node showing partial loss of architecture with widespread apoptosis and necrosis.

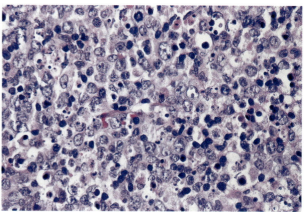

FIGURE 3.36 Kikuchi disease. Blast cells with numerous apoptotic bodies in the background.

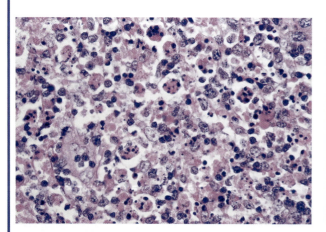

FIGURE 3.37 Kikuchi disease. An area of almost complete apoptosis and necrosis.

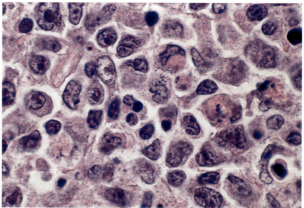

FIGURE 3.38 Kikuchi disease. High-power view showing blast cells and histiocytes with characteristic crescentic nuclei.

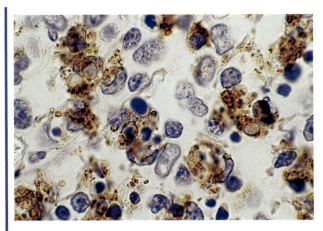

FIGURE 3.39 Kikuchi disease. Section stained for CD68, showing histiocytes with crescentic nuclei and phagocytosed apoptotic debris.

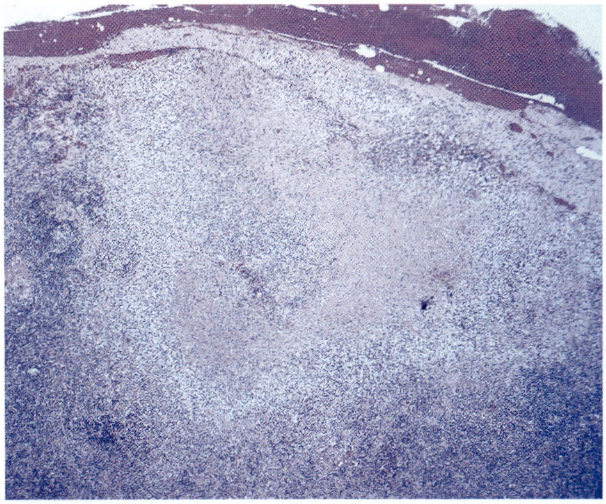

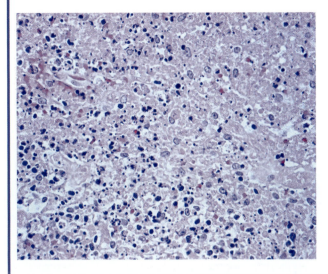

FIGURE 3.40 Systemic lupus erythematosus of lymph node showing a wedge-shaped area of subcapsular necrosis. The area of necrosis is less extensive than that usually seen in Kikuchi disease.

FIGURE 3.41 Higher power view of systemic lupus erythematosus of lymph node showing apoptosis and necrosis without polymorph infiltration.

BOX 3.13: Drug-induced lymphadenopathy

- History of exposure to drug, particularly anticonvulsant therapy
- Fever, skin rashes and lymphadenopathy
- Peripheral blood eosinophilia
- Paracortical expansion with mixed infiltrate including blast cells and eosinophils
- Small areas of necrosis may be present, often associated with eosinophils
- Regresses following drug withdrawal

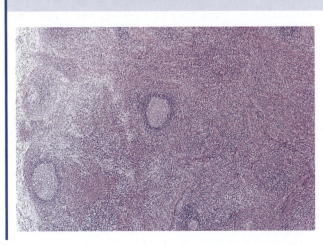

FIGURE 3.42 Drug-induced lymphadenopathy, showing reactive follicles and expanded paracortex.

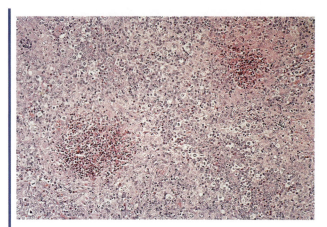

FIGURE 3.43 Drug-induced lymphadenopathy. Paracortex showing blast cell hyperplasia and eosinophil microabscesses.

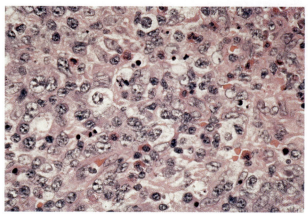

FIGURE 3.44 Drug-induced lymphadenopathy. High-power view of paracortex showing blast cells and eosinophils.

SINUS EXPANSION

SINUS HYPERPLASIA (SINUS HISTIOCYTOSIS)

Prominent sinuses containing many histiocytes are a feature seen in reactive lymph nodes, particularly from the mediastinum and the mesentery. This is often seen in lymph nodes draining carcinomas. The histiocytes do not show atypical features and other inflammatory cells may accompany them. Occasionally, the histiocytes contain oval bodies of variable size that have a green coloration in haematoxylin and eosin (H&E)-stained sections. These inclusions, known as Hamazaki–Wesenberg bodies, are composed of ceroid and are acid fast in Ziehl–Neelsen preparations. They probably result from the increased turnover of lipid membranes and should not be confused with organisms.

ROSAI–DORFMAN DISEASE (SINUS HISTIOCYTOSIS WITH MASSIVE LYMPHADENOPATHY)

This disease was first described in English by Rosai and Dorfman as sinus histiocytosis with massive lymphadenopathy. Since the disease may be extranodal as well as nodal, the use of the eponymous title is more appropriate. It may occur at all ages, but is most common in childhood and young adult life. There is a male predominance of 4:3.

Patients usually present with cervical lymphadenopathy, other lymph nodes being much less frequently involved. The lymphadenopathy is often massive and may be of long duration. Systemic symptoms of fever, night sweats, weight loss, malaise and arthralgia may be present. Laboratory tests often show hypochromic microcytic anaemia, hypergammaglobulinaemia and a raised erythrocyte sedimentation rate (ESR). The majority of cases undergo spontaneous regression or show persistent localized disease. A small number of patients have died, usually with more widespread disease. They often show evidence of immune deficiency.

Lymph nodes show varying degrees of capsular fibrosis. The most prominent histological feature is expansion of the sinuses that are filled with histiocytes. These characteristically have abundant, often vacuolated cytoplasm, and rounded nuclei with coarse chromatin and often a single prominent nucleolus. A proportion of these histiocytes show varying numbers of lymphocytes, which do not appear degenerate, within their cytoplasm. Less commonly, erythrocytes, plasma cells and polymorphs appear to be engulfed. The intervening medullary cords show large numbers of plasma cells. Residual reactive germinal centres may be seen but these regress with time. In long-standing cases, there is fibrous replacement of the involved nodes. This leads to persistence of the lymphadenopathy, and surgery may be needed for cosmetic reasons or to relieve obstruction.

A study using X-linked polymorphic loci has shown the histiocytes of Rosai–Dorfman disease to be polyclonal. The atypical histiocytes express CD68 and muramidase. In contrast to reactive sinus histiocytes, they are S100 positive, possibly indicating origin from antigen presenting cells. They are negative for CD1a.

Langerhans cell histiocytosis presenting as lymphadenopathy is uncommon and in this book has been included under 'Histiocytic and dendritic cell neoplasms' in Chapter 9 in keeping with the World Health Organization (WHO) classification. It is predominantly a sinus proliferation and thus enters into the differential diagnosis of Rosai–Dorfman disease. The histiocytes in the two diseases have different morphological characteristics. Both stain for S100 protein but only Langerhans cells express CD1a.

SINUS HISTIOCYTOSIS AND LIPOGRANULOMATOUS REACTION

Lipids of exogenous origin, such as parental nutrition fluids, contrast media used in lymphangiography, lipid-based substances and oils used as depot vehicles for the slow release of injected drugs, and endogenous lipids in patients who are obese, diabetic, hyperlipidemic or who have fat necrosis, haematomas or cholesterol deposits, may stimulate a lipogranulomatous reaction in lymph nodes.

Lipid granulomas are formed as a result of the accumulation histiocytes and foreign-body-type giant cells around lipid in the subcapsular and medullary sinuses. Phagocytosis of lipid by the macrophages and giant cells causes vacuolation of their cytoplasm. Epithelioid histiocytes may occur but they seldom aggregate to form discrete granulomas. Plasma cells, lymphocytes and sometimes eosinophils may accompany the histiocytic proliferation.

Lymph nodes at the porta hepatis

These nodes frequently show a lipogranulomatous reaction, often within the paracortex rather than in the sinuses.

Lymphangiogram effect

Haematopathologists became familiar with this reaction when staging laparotomies were performed as a part of the management of Hodgkin lymphoma. Lymphangiograms are now less frequently performed. The sinuses of the affected nodes are distended by a lipogranulomatous reaction to the oil-based contrast medium.

Silicone lymphadenopathy

Silicone in liquid form has been used for breast enhancement either by direct injection of silicone into the breast or by implanting a prosthesis containing silicone. The fluid causes a lipogranulomatous reaction followed by fibrosis in the breast and the draining lymph nodes.

Silicone in solid form causes a different type of lymphadenopathy. This is seen in patients who have received interphalangeal prostheses for severe rheumatoid arthritis. Small fragments of silicone carried to the lymph nodes causes a giant cell reaction in the sinuses or the paracortex. Refractile non-birefringent fragments of silicone are seen in these giant cells.

Infective causes

Whipple disease, a rare bacterial infection caused by *Tropheryma whippelii*, is associated with mesenteric lymphadenopathy but systemic lymphadenopathy is also seen in half the cases. Lipid vacuoles are characteristically present in the sinuses. The sinus histiocytes are distended by PAS-positive bacilli.

Numerous foamy histiocytes may be seen in lymph nodes from patients with lepromatous leprosy. These tend to be in the paracortex rather than in the sinuses. Ziehl–Neelsen stain shows numerous acid-fast leprosy bacilli.

Metabolic causes

Foamy macrophages are seen in Neimann–Pick and Fabry diseases. Genetic and biochemical tests are needed for their confirmation.

VASCULAR TRANSFORMATION OF SINUSES

This uncommon condition is most likely to be encountered in nodes removed at surgery for cancer. The cortical and medullary sinuses are filled with proliferating vascular channels of varying density. Vascular obstruction is thought to be the cause of this lesion, although angiogenic factors may play a role. The most important differential diagnosis is with Kaposi sarcoma. Kaposi sarcoma has a more solid structure, often involves the capsule and the blood-filled clefts between the spindle cells are not lined by endothelial cells.

BOX 3.14: Rosai–Dorfman disease

- Most common in childhood and young adult life
- Cervical lymphadenopathy most common presentation
- May occur at other nodal and extranodal sites
- Fever, night sweats, weight loss, malaise and arthralgia may occur
- Anaemia, hypergammaglobulinaemia and raised erythrocyte sedimentation rate (ESR) frequent

- Capsular fibrosis
- Sinuses expanded by histiocytes with rounded nuclei, prominent nucleoli and abundant cytoplasm
- Histiocytes engulf lymphocytes and other haematopoietic cells
- Large numbers of plasma cells in medullary cords

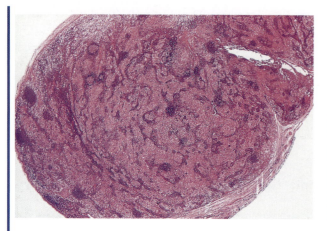

FIGURE 3.45 Rosai–Dorfman disease. Lymph node showing marked sinus histiocytosis with compression of other lymph node compartments.

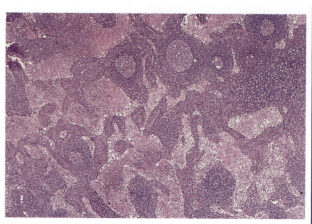

FIGURE 3.46 Rosai–Dorfman disease. Prominent sinus histiocytosis.

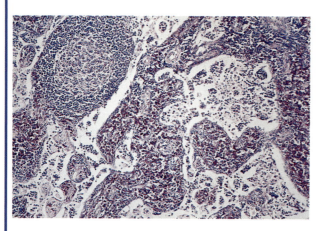

FIGURE 3.47 Rosai–Dorfman disease. Methyl-green pyronin-stained section. The medullary cords contain many pyroninophilic plasma cells. Note the lymphophagocytic histiocytes in the sinuses.

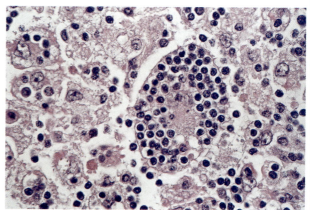

FIGURE 3.48 Rosai–Dorfman disease. High-power view showing lymphophagocytic histiocytes.

BOX 3.15: Lipogranulomatous lymphadenitis

- Exogenous lipid (lymphangiogram, parenteral nutrition)
- Endogenous lipid (obesity, diabetes, hyperlipidaemia)
- Sinus histiocytosis

- Sinuses contain lipid vacuoles surrounded by foamy histiocytes, giant cells and epithelioid cells
- Much of the lipid in nodes from the porta hepatis appears in the paracortex.

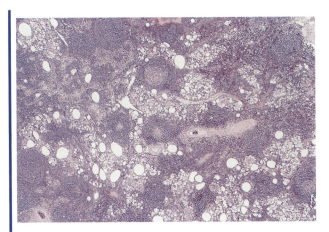

FIGURE 3.49 Lymph node from porta hepatis showing a lipogranulomatous reaction to lipid. Lipid vacuoles in the paracortex and sinuses are surrounded by histiocytes and giant cells.

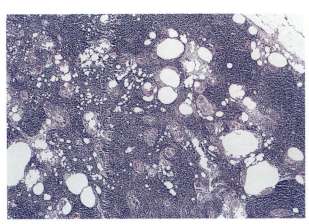

FIGURE 3.50 Lymphangiogram effect, para-aortic lymph node. The lipid-rich contrast medium has evoked a lipogranulomatous reaction in the lymph node sinuses.

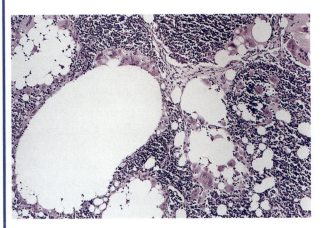

FIGURE 3.51 Lymphangiogram effect. High-power view showing histiocyte and giant cell reaction to the contrast medium.

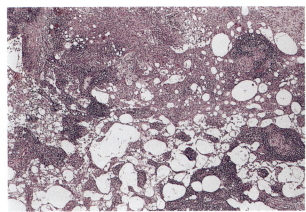

FIGURE 3.52 Whipple disease. The sinuses of the lymph node are filled with foamy histiocytes surrounding lipid vacuoles.

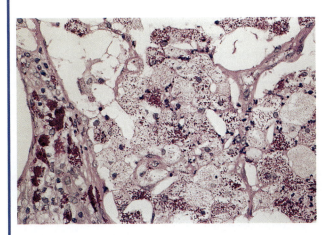

FIGURE 3.53 Whipple disease. Periodic acid Schiff stained section showing large numbers of bacilli in foamy histiocytes.

BOX 3.16: Vascular transformation of sinuses

- Most frequently encountered in lymph nodes draining carcinomas
- Probably due to vascular obstruction
- Proliferation of endothelial lined vascular spaces in subcapsular and medullary sinuses
- Sinuses often engorged with blood

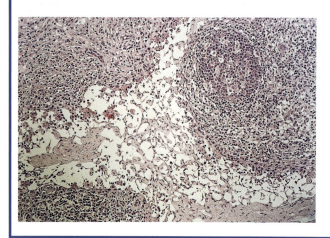

FIGURE 3.54 Vascular transformation of sinuses. The sinuses shown are filled with a meshwork of endothelial cell-lined vascular spaces.

GRANULOMATOUS LYMPHADENITIS

These are lymphadenopathies that are characterized by the presence of granulomas or localized aggregates of histiocytes as the most prominent feature. They may be conveniently divided into those with suppuration (i.e. necrosis and the presence of neutrophils) and those granulomas formed of epithelioid histiocytes. The latter group may be further divided into non-necrotizing or sarcoid-like granulomatous, and necrotizing granulomatous lymphadenitis. All groups of reaction however, may be accompanied by varying degrees of follicular and paracortical hyperplasia but the granulomatous reaction is the most prominent feature.

SUPPURATIVE GRANULOMATOUS LYMPHADENOPATHY

Suppurative granulomatous lymphadenitis generally represents a B-cell-associated granulomatous reaction that is different from the hypersensitivity type or epithelioid granulomatous lymphadenitis seen in tuberculosis, leprosy and sarcoidosis. Suppurative granulomas often appear to start as an accumulation of monocytoid B-cells followed by polymorph infiltration with necrosis developing in these foci, leading eventually to granuloma formation. This contrasts with the formation of epithelioid granulomas of the hypersensitivity-type, which appears to be mediated by activated T-cells, dendritic cells and histiocytes without the

participation of B-cells. Suppurative granulomas are distinguished from the hypersensitivity-type granulomas by the presence of neutrophils, prominence of monocytoid B-cells and a paucity of multinucleated giant cells. Immunostaining reveals a mixture of B- and T-cells mixed with histiocytes, polymorphs, immunoblasts and dendritic cells. In contrast, B-cells are few or absent within hypersensitivity-type granulomas.

Included among the more common causes of bacterial suppurative granulomatous lymphadenitis are cat scratch disease, lymphogranuloma venereum, tularaemia and *Yersinia* infections (Box 3.17). There are no specific morphological features to distinguish between these various entities and they will be described together.

BOX 3.17: Common aetiologic agents in suppurative granulomatous lymphadenopathy

Bartonella henselae (cat scratch disease)
Chlamydia trachomatis (lymphogranuloma venereum)
Francisella tularensis (tularaemia)
Yersinia enterocolitica, Y. pseudotuberculosis
Listeria monocytogenes
Pseudomonas mallei (glanders), *P. pseudomallei* (melioidosis)
Corynebacterium ovis, C. pyogenes, C. ulcerans

The demonstration of the causative agent by histochemical and/or immunohistochemical stains and the use of serological tests, bacterial culture or molecular techniques such as polymerase chain reaction (PCR) provides the definitive aetiological diagnosis.

The lymph nodes involved are generally regional nodes draining the portal of entry of the causative organism but systemic dissemination may occur with progression of the infection. There is initially a florid follicular hyperplasia with abundant monocytoid B-cells in the sinuses and parafollicular areas while nodal architecture remains preserved. Subsequently, small suppurative granulomas develop. These comprise collections of histiocytes with and without central aggregates of neutrophils, and occur in close proximity to the monocytoid B-cell clusters from which they may be difficult to separate. In later stages there is coalescence of the enlarging granulomas, which display central stellate areas of necrosis that contain neutrophil debris (nuclear dust) and fibrinoid material, and are surrounded by a rim of palisading histiocytes, often with proliferating fibroblasts. The monocytoid B-cells may be less prominent at this stage. Multinucleated cells are rare.

Cat scratch disease

The causative organism of cat scratch disease is *Bartonella henselae*, a Gram-positive pleomorphic coccobacillus that can be found in clumps in the foci of necrosis and around blood vessels and within sinusoidal macrophages, especially in the late phase of the disease. The organisms can be demonstrated in over 60 per cent of cases with the Warthin–Starry stain or Dieterle stain, or immunohistochemically. Cat scratch disease is the most common cause of suppurative granulomatous lymphadenitis and may show systemic involvement including suppurative hepatosplenic granulomas and osteomyelitis.

Lymphogranuloma venereum

Lymphogranuloma venereum may show vacuolated macrophages containing *Chlamydia trachomatis*, as fine, sand-like infective organisms, in and around the suppurative areas, as demonstrated with the Warthin–Starry stain. There is often accompanying oedema with inflammation around the lymph node (perilymphadenitis).

Yersinia lymphadenitis

Yersinia lymphadenitis shows no distinguishing features from the other forms of suppurative granulomatous lymphadenitis other than its mesenteric location and may be associated with changes in the terminal ileum. Confirmation requires culture or serological testing.

Other causes of suppurative granulomatous lymphadenitis

Tularaemia, caused by *Francisella tularensis*, is transmitted by ticks and other biting arthropods, produces a necrotizing granulomatous lymphadenitis that is indistinguishable from the preceding diseases and may be associated with Langhans-type giant cells. Other rare causes of suppurative granulomatous lymphadenitis include infection by *Listeria monocytogenes*, *Pseudomonas mallei* (glanders) and *Pseudomonas pseudomallei* (melioidosis), which cannot be distinguished except by identification of the causative organism in the tissue section, culture or PCR. *Corynebacteria*, especially *ovis*, *ulcerans*, *diphtheriae* and *pyogenes* can produce suppurative granulomas in draining lymph nodes.

EPITHELIOID GRANULOMATOUS LYMPHADENOPATHY (HYPERSENSITIVITY-TYPE GRANULOMATOSIS)

The common causes of epithelioid or hypersensitivity-type granulomatous lymphadenopathy are listed in Box 3.18. They may be divided into necrotizing and non-necrotizing groups, with tuberculosis and sarcoidosis, respectively, representing the prototypes of these two reactions.

BOX 3.18: Common causes of epithelioid granulomatous lymphadenitis

NECROTIZING GRANULOMAS
Mycobacteria tuberculosis, M. avium intracellulare, M. lepra
Systemic fungal infections, especially *Cryptococcus neoformans, Histoplasma capsulatum, Coccidioides immitis, Blastomycosis dermatitidis*

NON-NECROTIZING GRANULOMAS
Sarcoidosis
Berylliosis
Crohn's disease
Lymph nodes draining carcinoma

Necrotizing epithelioid granulomatous lymphadenopathy

Tuberculous lymphadenitis

Tuberculous lymphadenitis is the prototype of necrotizing epithelioid granulomatous lymphadenitis with central areas of caseous necrosis surrounded by palisaded epithelioid histiocytes and Langhans giant cells. Variable numbers of T-cells are found around the palisading epithelioid cells. Proliferating fibroblasts may be present around the entire granuloma. There is a tendency for tuberculous granulomas to coalesce forming confluent areas of necrosis and granulomatous inflammation. Tubercle bacilli demonstrated with the Ziehl–Neelsen stain may be difficult to find; they are usually most easily detected within the necrotic areas or in the cytoplasm of giant cells. Other mycobacteria including *Mycobacterium scrofulaceum*, *bovis*, *kansasii*, *marinum*, *ulcerans*, and *fortuitum* can produce a similar appearing lymphadenitis, as can bacillus Calmette–Guérin (BCG).

Mycobacterium avium-intracellulare may produce an indistinguishable necrotizing granulomatous response but may also show a wide spectrum of histological changes that include a striking histiocytosis with a spindle-cell proliferation of short fascicles and a storiform pattern that may be mistaken for fibrous histiocytoma, inflammatory pseudotumour or smooth muscle tumour. In all these reactions, the atypical mycobacteria are readily demonstrated with a Ziehl–Neelsen, methenamine silver, PAS or Gram stain. The stains may often reveal myriads of bacilli similar to the globi of lepromatous leprosy that can be seen as basophilic cytoplasmic streaks in H&E sections.

In tuberculoid leprosy, the nodes show discrete epithelioid granulomas with a variable number of Langhans giant cells but without necrosis. The granulomas may undergo fibrosis and hyalinization, and may mimic sarcoidosis. The lepromatous form of the disease gives rise to a striking paracortical histiocytosis with large clusters of the bacilli or globi within the foam cells, also called lepra cells or Virchow cells. In borderline leprosy, the nodal morphology may be either that of the tuberculoid or lepromatous disease.

Fungal lymphadenopathy

Fungal infections of lymph nodes can be divided into primary and opportunistic infections, the latter infecting immune-compromised patients. This division is somewhat artificial, as even the primary or deep mycoses require some degree of depression of immunity to produce systemic infection. Fungal infections may result in a spectrum of changes ranging from histiocytosis to epithelioid granulomas with or without suppurative necrosis and the specific diagnosis is based on identification of the fungus by special stains or culture. The following systemic mycotic infections can involve lymph nodes: cryptococcosis (*Cryptococcus neoformans*), histoplasmosis (*Histoplasma capsulatum*), coccidioidomycosis (*Coccidioides immitis*) and blastomycosis (*Blastomyces dermatitidis*).

Lymph node involvement in cryptococcosis occurs most commonly in mediastinal nodes secondary to pulmonary infections. The extent of granulomatous reaction is very variable, ranging from minimal cellular reaction to full-blown granulomas, but the yeast-like organisms are often numerous. They are refractile, of variable size, and have a clear halo around the cell wall. This halo represents the mucopolysaccharide capsule, which is demonstrated by PAS or Grocott stains.

Nodal involvement by histoplasmosis generally follows pulmonary infection and shows pathological features that resemble tuberculosis. The enlarged nodes contain tuberculoid granulomas and often undergo caseous necrosis. The necrotic areas are frequently surrounded by a fibrous reaction and may calcify. The histological reaction in patients with HIV/AIDS and other forms of immunodeficiency lacks granuloma formation. Sheets of histiocytes containing numerous organisms replace the lymph node. The encapsulated budding yeasts are best visualized with the Grocott or PAS stain within the areas of necrosis, and within histiocytes and giant cells.

Other pathogenic fungi produce a range of cellular responses. In some situations, the lymph node reaction may be non-specific, especially in nodes draining infected sites where a non-specific germinal centre and paracortical hyperplasia are seen without granuloma formation. Although many fungi are visible in H&E-stained sections, the PAS and Grocott stains allow better visualization of the organism and, whenever fungal lymphadenitis is suspected, fungal culture should be performed.

Non-necrotizing granulomatous lymphadenopathy

Sarcoidosis

The granulomas of sarcoidosis are composed of clusters of epithelioid histiocytes with occasional giant cells surrounded by variable numbers of T-cells. They show a lesser tendency than tuberculous granulomas to coalesce and do not show caseous necrosis, although small areas of central necrosis may be seen. The mult-inucleated giant cells may contain birefringent rounded concretions known as Schaumann bodies. Calcium and iron can be demonstrated in these layered inclusions. Less frequently asteroid bodies are present. These are inclusions with varying numbers of curved processes radiating from the centre. While striking in appearance, neither of these inclusions is specific and may be found in other reactive conditions. With disease progression the granulomas become surrounded by, and are eventually replaced by, fibrous tissue.

Berylliosis

The granulomatous lymphadenitis caused by beryllium is histologically indistinguishable from sarcoid.

Protozoan and nematode infections

Lymphadenitis caused by protozoa, nematodes, larval nematodes and ova are generally uncommon and represent more a curiosity; however, in endemic areas, this form of lymph node involvement may be routinely encountered. These infections are discussed under granulomatous reactions because they do not conform to any specific reaction pattern and a granulomatous response is the most common reaction to the parasitic antigens. Follicular hyperplasia may also be present and eosinophilia is a frequent accompaniment of such infections.

Lymphadenitis due to Entamoeba histolytica

Amoebiasis caused by *Entamoeba histolytica* may involve lymph nodes with the protozoa being carried to draining lymph nodes. As the amoebae closely mimic the appearance of foamy macrophages and even carcinoma cells, and as they tend to be located in the sinuses in the first instance, they should not be mistaken for these cells. Both macrophages and amoebae may contain ingested red cells and may be positive with PAS-stain but the amoebae also stain with colloidal iron. Carcinoma cells are readily excluded on the basis of immunostaining for cytokeratin.

Leishmania *lymphadenitis*

The protozoan *Leishmania* sp. is endemic in many areas of the world, where it is transmitted by sandflies. Ulcers may develop at the site of sandfly bites. Local lymph nodes are frequently involved and lymphadenopathy may be the presenting feature. Disseminated disease gives rise to visceral leishmaniasis (kala-azar) and is also seen in HIV/AIDS patients.

Lymph nodes show reactive changes, with loose collections of histiocytes in the paracortex. As the disease progresses, these become more organized as epithelioid giant cell granulomas. In the early stages of the disease and in immunodeficient individuals, the parasite amastigotes are easily found within histiocytes. When well-formed granulomas are present, it is often not possible to find organisms, although they are detectable by PCR.

Lymphadenitis due to metazoan parasites

Metazoan parasites may occasionally be found in lymph nodes. Among these are *Ascaris lumbricoides*, the common roundworm, *Toxocara catti* and *Toxocara canis* (cat and dog ascarid), *Strongyloides stercoralis*, *Ancylostoma duodenale*, *Necator americanus* (hookworms), *Trichinella spiralis* (pork worm), *Oxyuris vermicularis* (threadworm), *Trichuris trichura* (whipworm) and *Wuchereria bancrofti* (filariasis), *Brugia melayi* (filariasis), *Onchocerca volvulus* (river blindness) and *Dracunculus medinensis* (Guinea worm). The adult and larval forms of these nematodes may enter blood vessels and lymphatics during their migration. When they lodge in the lymph node and die, they produce a granulomatous reaction, often with the nematode in the centre. Invariably, there is accompanying necrosis and multinucleated giant cells, eosinophils and the Splendore–Hoeppli reaction may occur around the dead nematode. This granulomatous reaction is eventually replaced by fibrosis, which may cause lymphatic obstruction and lymphoedema.

Lymph nodes draining malignancy

Lymph nodes draining malignancy, most frequently carcinoma, may show a sarcoid-like granulomatous response in the absence of tumour deposits in the node. Such epithelioid granulomas are seen in a variety of carcinomas and are the result of stimulation by antigens from the tumour carried to the regional nodes.

Lymphadenopathy due to foreign materials

Detritic lymphadenitis is a granulomatous reaction to the cementing material and metallic debris that migrate from joint prosthesis to draining lymph nodes. The flakes of foreign material are pigmented and the cementing substances are both birefringent and refractile, and are present in macrophages within the sinuses and paracortex.

Tattoo pigment is usually seen in the paracortex of nodes draining an area of tattooing. Black granules are seen in macrophages. Careful examination of this pigment will usually reveal other red, green and blue pigments. These are often birefringent and are highlighted by visualization in polarized light. Tattoo pigment is sometimes associated with areas of necrosis and/or granuloma formation, presumably resulting from hypersensitivity to one of the components.

BOX 3.19: Suppurative granulomatous lymphadenitis

- Usually involves lymph nodes draining the portal of entry of the causative organism
- Follicular hyperplasia
- Monocytoid B-cell hyperplasia with a variable infiltrate of polymorphs
- Areas of necrosis develop, surrounded by palisaded histiocytes but few giant cells
- Areas of necrosis assume a serpiginous or stellate shape
- Aetiologic agent may be demonstrated by special stains, culture or the polymerase chain reaction

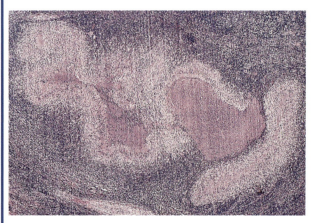

FIGURE 3.55 Cat scratch disease. Lymph node showing serpiginous areas of necrosis surrounded by palisaded epithelioid histiocytes.

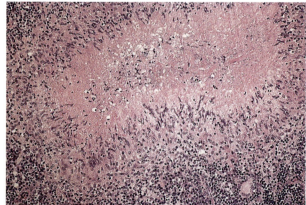

FIGURE 3.56 Cat scratch disease. High-power view showing palisaded epithelioid histiocytes around an area of necrosis. Some of the nuclear debris at the centre of the area of necrosis is from polymorph leucocytes.

BOX 3.20: Epithelioid granulomatous lymphadenopathy

- Histological appearances vary from loose collections of epithelioid cells or solitary giant cells to well-formed granulomas
- Histological appearance varies with the causative agent and the host's immune status
- Special stains (periodic acid Schiff, Grocott, Ziehl–Neelsen and Giemsa) aid the identification of many organisms.

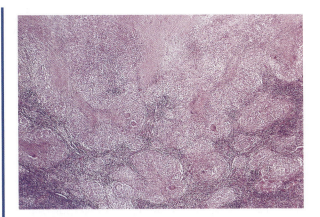

FIGURE 3.57 Tuberculous lymph node showing necrotizing epithelioid cell/giant cell granulomas. Note the tendency of the granulomas to coalesce.

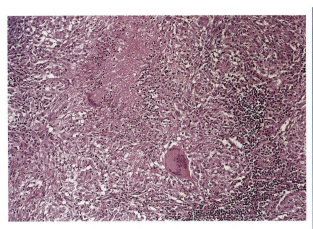

FIGURE 3.58 Tuberculous lymph node showing caseating granulomas containing Langhans-type giant cells.

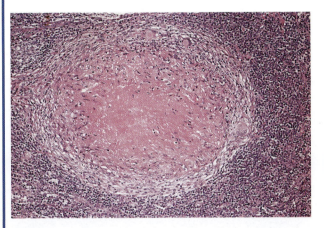

FIGURE 3.59 Bacille Calmette–Guérin (BCG)-infected lymph node from an immunocompetent patient showing a well-defined necrotizing granuloma.

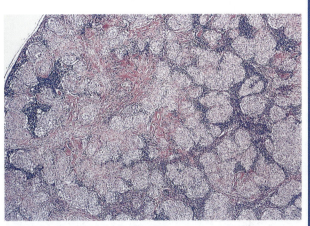

FIGURE 3.60 Sarcoidosis of lymph node. The granulomas tend to remain discrete and to undergo progressive fibrosis.

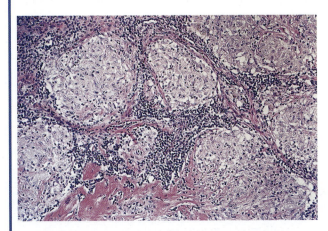

FIGURE 3.61 Sarcoidosis of lymph node showing well-defined non-necrotizing epithelioid cell granulomas undergoing early sclerosis.

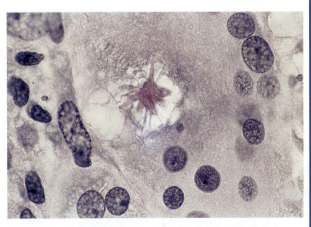

FIGURE 3.62 Sarcoidosis of lymph node showing an asteroid body in a giant cell.

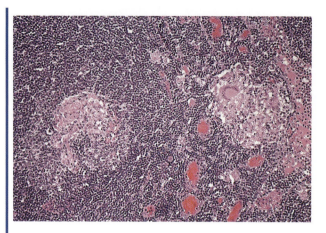

FIGURE 3.63 Abdominal lymph node from a patient with Crohn's disease showing two granulomas.

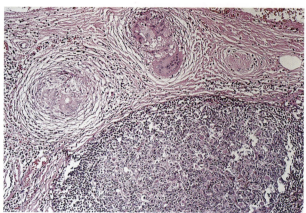

FIGURE 3.64 Lymph node from a patient with schistosomiasis. There is marked capsular fibrosis with several granulomas surrounding schistosome ova.

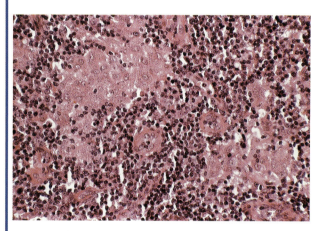

FIGURE 3.65 Leishmaniasis of lymph node. Organisms are visible in the cytoplasm of the histiocytes.

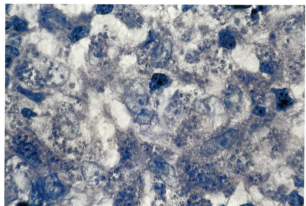

FIGURE 3.66 Leishmaniasis of lymph node, Giemsa stain. The organisms are seen more easily with this stain than with haematoxylin and eosin.

BOX 3.21: Infective lymphadenopathy in patients with impaired or absent immune response

- Sheets of histiocytes without well-defined granuloma formation
- Histiocytes have abundant eosinophilic or foamy cytoplasm
- Large numbers of organisms demonstrable within the histiocytes
- Areas of necrosis may occur within the histiocyte aggregates

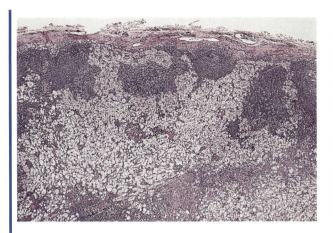

FIGURE 3.67 Lepromatous leprosy. Foamy histiocytes (lepra cells) fill the paracortex of the node.

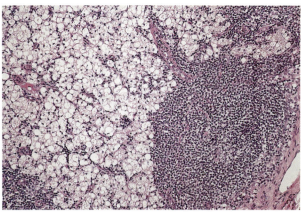

FIGURE 3.68 Lepromatous leprosy. High-power view of lepra cells.

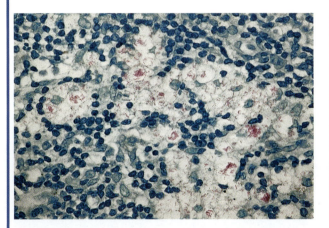

FIGURE 3.69 Lepromatous leprosy. Stain for acid-fast bacilli shows large numbers of leprosy bacilli in lepra cells.

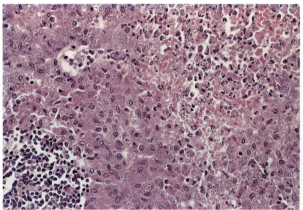

FIGURE 3.70 Bacille Calmette–Guérin (BCG)-infected lymph node from an immunosuppressed patient showing an area of necrosis surrounded by plump histiocytes.

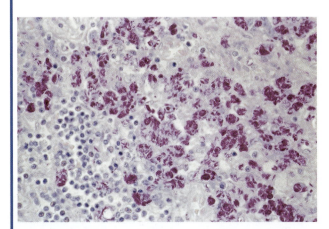

FIGURE 3.71 Bacille Calmette–Guérin (BCG)-infected lymph node from an immunosuppressed patient stained by the Ziehl–Neelsen method. Large numbers of acid-fast bacilli fill the plump histiocytes.

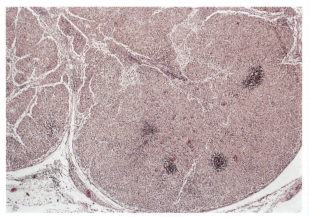

FIGURE 3.72 *Mycobacterium avium intracellulare* infection in an immunosuppressed patient. Sheets of pale-staining histiocytes replace the lymph node.

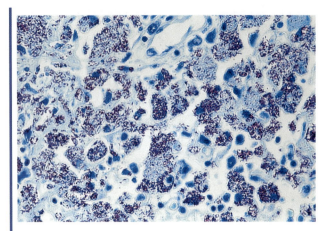

FIGURE 3.73 *Mycobacterium avium intracellulare* infection. Ziehl–Neelsen-stained section, showing histiocytes filled with acid-fast bacilli.

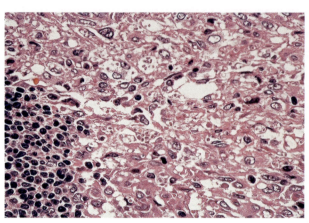

FIGURE 3.74 Histoplasmosis. Clusters of yeasts are seen within the cytoplasm of histiocytes.

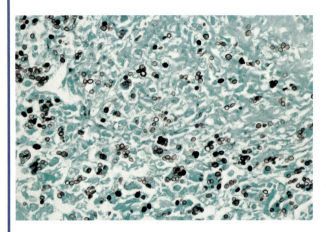

FIGURE 3.75 Histoplasmosis. Grocott stain highlights the intracellular organisms.

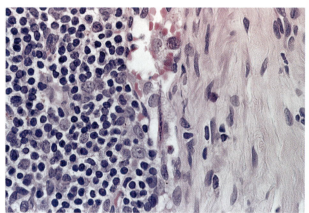

FIGURE 3.76 Lymph node from a patient with onchocerciasis. There is fibrosis of the capsule and a microfilaria is seen in the subcapsular sinus. Since the organism was alive at the time of biopsy, it has not excited a granulomatous reaction.

BOX 3.22: Lymphadenopathy due to foreign materials

- Reaction to inhaled, injected or implanted foreign materials
- Commonly encountered causes include tattoo pigment and debris from joint prostheses
- Material may be pigmented
- Material may be birefringent

- There may be no reaction to the foreign material
- Reaction may take the form of epithelioid cell giant cell granulomas or of foreign-body-type giant cells
- Necrosis may be present

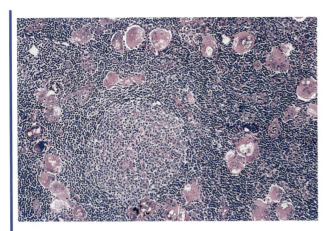

FIGURE 3.77 Silicone lymphadenopathy. This paracortical giant cell reaction is to particulate silicone from a joint prosthesis.

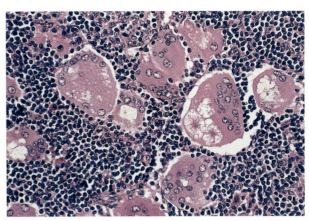

FIGURE 3.78 Silicone lymphadenopathy. High-power view showing asteroid bodies and refractile silicone particles in the giant cells.

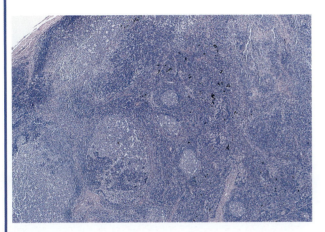

FIGURE 3.79 Tattoo pigment in a hyperplastic lymph node. The pigment is mainly distributed in the paracortex.

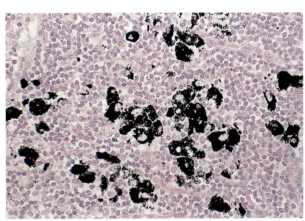

FIGURE 3.80 Tattoo pigment in paracortical histiocytes. Carbon is the main black pigment but other colours are seen.

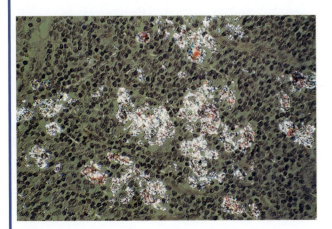

FIGURE 3.81 Tattoo pigment viewed in polarized light showing multiple colours.

PRECURSOR B- AND T-CELL LYMPHOMAS

PRECURSOR B-LYMPHOBLASTIC LEUKAEMIA/LYMPHOBLASTIC LYMPHOMA

B-Lymphoblastic leukaemia and B-lymphoblastic lymphoma are essentially one disease process. Those patients with predominantly blood and bone marrow involvement are designated as leukaemia; those with nodal or extranodal disease and less than 25 per cent lymphoblasts in the bone marrow are designated as lymphoma. In practice, the majority of cases are leukaemic. Although B-lymphoblastic leukaemia/lymphoma is approximately four times as common as T-lymphoblastic leukaemia/lymphoma, the T-cell neoplasms present more frequently as a solid tumour (lymphoma).

B-Lymphoblastic lymphoma presents most commonly as skin nodules, often multiple, bone tumours and lymphadenopathy. The tumour occurs most commonly in childhood with fewer young adult cases.

Morphologically, B-lymphoblastic and T-lymphoblastic lymphoma are indistinguishable. The tumour is composed of medium-sized blast cells that may be very uniform or show varying degrees of anisocytosis. Nuclei may be rounded or convoluted. The latter feature is best seen in imprints, very thin sections or plastic-embedded tissue. Convoluted nuclei do not have any phenotypic or clinical significance. In formalin-fixed tissues, the nuclear chromatin appears smooth or like fine dust. Nucleoli are usually small and inconspicuous. Mitotic figures are usually easily seen. The cytoplasm shows only weak basophilia in Giemsa-stained preparations and is indistinct in haematoxylin and eosin (H&E)-stained sections.

Lymphoblastic lymphomas infiltrate lymph nodes in the manner of a leukaemia leaving the reticulin structure relatively intact and often leaving isolated germinal centres. Where the tumour cells infiltrate the capsule, hilum and around blood vessels, they often adopt an Indian file formation between connective tissue fibres. Scattered histiocytes may give the tumour a 'starry-sky' appearance, but this is never as prominent as in Burkitt lymphoma and the histiocytes contain less apoptotic debris.

IMMUNOHISTOCHEMISTRY

Many B-lymphoblastic lymphomas do not express CD45 detectable in paraffin sections, a potential pitfall for the unwary in the differential diagnosis of small blue cell tumours. Similarly, many cases do not express CD20. The most reliable B-cell marker expressed on B-lymphoblastic lymphoma is CD79a, although it should be noted that this is also expressed by many T-lymphoblastic lymphomas. Conversely, B-lymphoblastic lymphoma does not express T-cell antigens, although CD43 (sometimes erroneously considered to be a T-cell specific antigen) labels B-lymphoblastic lymphoma. Most cases of B-lymphoblastic lymphoma express CD10; CD34 labels about half of the cases. The precursor status of B-lymphoblastic lymphoma is established by positive nuclear staining for terminal deoxynucleotidyl transferase (TdT).

GENETICS

The majority of cases of B-lymphoblastic lymphoma show clonal, but unmutated, rearrangements of the immunoglobulin genes. Of these, two-thirds show clonal immunoglobulin heavy chain (IgH) rearrangements, and two-thirds show clonally rearranged IgH and light chain genes. A total of 60–80 per cent of cases also show T-cell receptor (TCR) gene rearrangements.

The cytogenetic abnormalities detected in B-lymphoblastic leukaemia/lymphoma (mainly established on leukaemic cases) are varied and have prognostic significance. The two commonest abnormalities, together accounting for more than half of all cases, are t(12;21) and hyperdiploidy, usually with trisomy of chromosomes 4 and 10, and have a favourable prognosis. The Philadelphia chromosomal abnormality t(9;22) occurs in a small number of cases of B-lymphoblastic leukaemia.

DIFFERENTIAL DIAGNOSIS

B-Lymphoblastic lymphoma cannot be distinguished from T-lymphoblastic lymphoma on morphology alone. Clinical features may help in that T-lymphoblastic lymphoma patients frequently have mediastinal (thymic) tumours, a rare feature in B-lymphoblastic lymphoma. Immunohistochemical profiles will usually separate the two entities. B-Lymphoblastic lymphoma expresses CD79a but not CD3, whereas T-lymphoblastic lymphoma may express CD79a but also expresses CD3. Gene rearrangement studies show clonal Ig heavy and/or light chain rearrangements in B-lymphoblastic lymphoma but may also show rearrangement of one or more of the TCR genes. T-Lymphoblastic lymphoma shows clonal rearrangement of the TCR genes but may show IgH rearrangements in 10–25 per cent of cases.

Myeloid sarcoma may mimic lymphoblastic lymphoma. It can often be identified by the presence of granulated cells. The expression of myelomonocytic markers on these tumours can usually be demonstrated by immunohistochemistry.

The blastoid variant of mantle cell lymphoma may closely resemble lymphoblastic lymphoma and probably

---

▲ BOX 4.1: B-Lymphoblastic lymphoma: clinical features

- ▲ Predominantly a childhood disease with occasional adult patients
- ▲ Common sites of involvement are skin, bone and lymph nodes
- ▲ Central nervous system and testes are common sites of relapse
- ▲ Designated as lymphoblastic leukaemia, if the bone marrow contains more than 25 per cent lymphoblasts

---

● BOX 4.2: Lymphoblastic lymphoma: morphology

- Infiltrates lymph node leaving reticulin architecture partially intact
- Residual reactive germinal centres may be present
- Infiltration of capsule and around blood vessels often shows Indian file pattern

- Smooth or dust-like nuclear chromatin
- Inconspicuous nucleoli
- Cytoplasm inconspicuous
- Nuclei may be convoluted
- Mitotic figures frequent

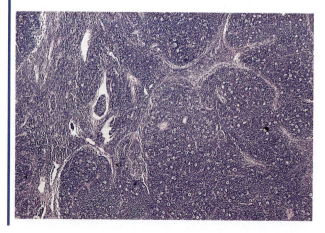

FIGURE 4.1 Low-power photograph of lymphoblastic lymphoma. Note preservation of much of the underlying nodal structure. Numerous 'starry-sky' macrophages are seen in this tumour.

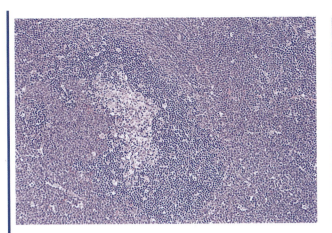

FIGRUE 4.2 Lymphoblastic lymphoma. The uniform tumour cells surround and partially invade a residual reactive follicle.

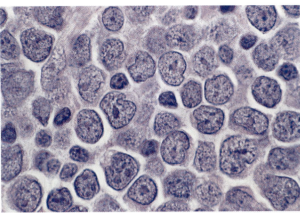

FIGURE 4.3 High-power view of lymphoblastic lymphoma. The tumour cells are relatively uniform in size, have fine nuclear chromatin and show one or more small nucleoli.

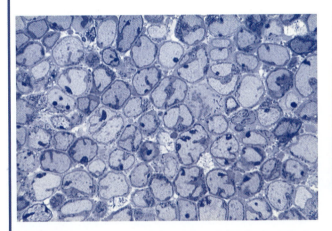

FIGURE 4.4 Plastic-embedded section of lymphoblastic lymphoma showing deep fissuring of the tumour cell nuclei, a feature seen in some but not all cases.

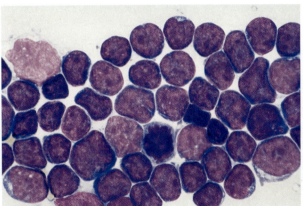

FIGURE 4.5 Imprint preparation of lymphoblastic lymphoma showing uniform size of tumour cells, fine nuclear chromatin and multiple nucleoli. The cytoplasmic rim is narrow and inconspicuous on most cells.

◆ BOX 4.3: B-Lymphoblastic lymphoma: immunohistochemistry

- ◆ Often CD45 negative
- ◆ Often CD20 negative
- ◆ CD79a positive, CD3 negative
- ◆ CD10 positive
- ◆ CD43 positive
- ◆ CD34 positive in 50 per cent of cases
- ◆ Terminal deoxynucleotidyl transferase (TdT) positive

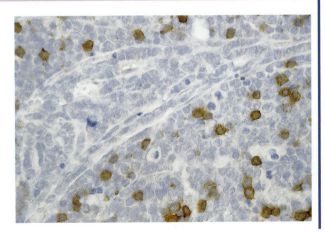

FIGURE 4.6 B-Lymphoblastic lymphoma stained for CD20. Reactive B-lymphocytes show positivity; the tumour cells are negative.

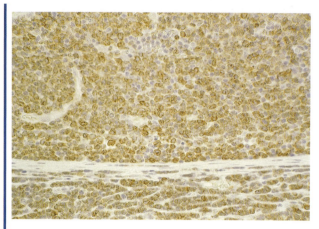

FIGURE 4.7 B-Lymphoblastic lymphoma stained for CD79a. The tumour cells are positive. Note 'Indian file' arrangement of the cells outside the capsule.

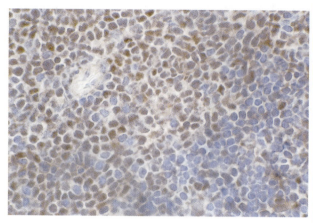

FIGURE 4.8 Lymphoblastic lymphoma stained for terminal deoxynucleotidyl transferase (TdT). The lymphoma cells show nuclear positivity. Residual mantle B-cells are negative.

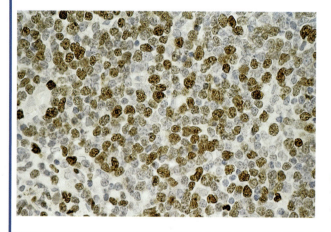

FIGURE 4.9 Lymphoblastic lymphoma stained for Ki67. The proliferation fraction in this tumour is in the region of 70 per cent.

accounts for many of the cases of adult lymphoblastic lymphoma reported in the past. Immunohistochemistry will clearly separate the two entities, with lymphoblastic lymphoma being TdT positive and mantle cell lymphoma cyclin-D1 positive.

Burkitt lymphoma (BL) has in the past been confused with lymphoblastic lymphoma and leukaemic cases were included in the French–American–British (FAB) classification of lymphoblastic lymphomas. Morphologically,

BL cells have granular nuclear chromatin and show intense cytoplasmic basophilia. They exhibit a mature B-cell phenotype and are TdT negative.

Rarely, diffuse large B-cell lymphoma will come into the differential diagnosis of lymphoblastic lymphoma, if the tumour cells appear small and have smooth chromatin with inconspicuous nucleoli. As with BL, these will exhibit a mature B-cell phenotype and will not express TdT.

PRECURSOR T-LYMPHOBLASTIC LEUKAEMIA/LYMPHOBLASTIC LYMPHOMA

Leukaemia and lymphoma are regarded as two related facets of precursor T-lymphoblastic neoplasia. T-lymphoblastic neoplasia is less common than B-lymphoblastic neoplasia, but a larger proportion of patients present with solid tumours and without evidence of leukaemia. The arbitrary cut-off point for leukaemia, as with B-lymphoblastic neoplasia, is less than 25 per cent

bone marrow lymphoblasts. T-Lymphoblastic lymphoma occurs at an older age than B-lymphoblastic lymphoma and is more frequent in males. The peak incidence is in adolescent males.

Anterior mediastinal (thymic) tumours are common in T-lymphoblastic lymphoma/leukaemia; they often cause mediastinal obstruction and may be associated with pleural effusions. Lymph nodes and extranodal sites may be involved. The central nervous system and gonads may be involved at presentation, and are common sites of relapse.

Morphologically, T-lymphoblastic lymphoma is indistinguishable from B-lymphoblastic lymphoma. It is composed of medium-sized blast cells that infiltrate lymph nodes, leaving much of the underlying reticulin structure intact. Infiltration into connective tissue structures often shows an Indian file pattern. Tumour cell nuclei may be rounded or convoluted with fine nuclear chromatin and small inconspicuous nucleoli. The mitotic index is usually high. The tumour cell cytoplasm is weakly basophilic in Giemsa-stained preparations and not clearly defined in H&E-stained sections. Scattered histiocytes giving a 'starry-sky' pattern may be present.

IMMUNOHISTOCHEMISTRY

T-Lymphoblastic lymphoma shows variable expression of CD1a, CD2, CD3, CD4, CD5, CD7 and CD8. Of these, CD3 is the most frequently expressed and is the most reliable lineage marker. CD43 is positive and myeloid associated antigens may be expressed. T-Lymphoblastic lymphoma may express CD10, and CD79a is weakly positive in almost half the biopsies. All cases are TdT positive.

GENETICS

T-Lymphoblastic leukaemia/lymphoma usually demonstrates clonal rearrangement of one or more of the T-cell receptor genes but, since these occur with high frequency in B-lymphoblastic leukaemia/lymphoma, they are not lineage specific. About one-third of cases show translocations between one of the T-cell receptor genes and a number of oncogenes. Loss of 9p occurs in about one-third of the cases resulting in loss of the tumour suppressor gene CDKN2A. The *TAL-1* gene involved in haematopoietic growth control is dysregulated by deletions in its regulatory region in 25 per cent of cases.

DIFFERENTIAL DIAGNOSIS

T-Lymphoblastic lymphoma and B-lymphoblastic lymphoma are indistinguishable morphologically, although they show clinical differences. They also show overlap in their immunohistochemical profile, with many T-lymphoblastic lymphomas weakly expressing CD79a. The most reliable distinguishing marker is CD3, expressed only on T-lymphoblastic lymphoma.

An uncommon variant of myeloid leukaemia in lymphoid blast crisis may mimic T-lymphoblastic lymphoma. These cases are associated with t(8;13)(p11.2; q11–22). Morphologically, the infiltrate resembles lymphoblastic lymphoma, but also contains granulated promyelocytes and myelocytes. The appearance thus mimics myeloid sarcoma, except that the non-granulated blasts express CD3. Most cases progress to acute myeloid leukaemia.

> ### ▲ BOX 4.4: T-Lymphoblastic lymphoma: clinical features
>
> ▲ Childhood and young adult disease with a peak incidence in adolescence
> ▲ Male predominance
> ▲ Involves anterior mediastinum most frequently. May cause mediastinal obstruction and be associated with pleural effusions
> ▲ Also involves lymph nodes, liver, spleen and skin
> ▲ Central nervous system and testes are common sites of relapse
> ▲ Designated as lymphoblastic leukaemia if the bone marrow lymphoblasts exceed 25 per cent

> ### ● BOX 4.5: T-Lymphoblastic lymphoma: morphology
>
> See box 4.2.

> ### ◆ BOX 4.6: T-Lymphoblastic lymphoma: immunohistochemistry
>
> ◆ Variable expression of CD1a, CD2, CD3, CD4, CD5, CD7 and CD8
> ◆ CD3 is most frequently expressed and is the most reliable lineage marker
> ◆ CD43 positive
> ◆ May express some myeloid antigens
> ◆ May express CD10
> ◆ Many cases express CD79a
> ◆ Terminal deoxynucleotidyl transferase (TdT) always positive

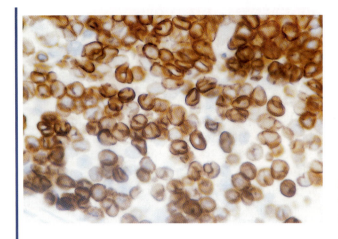

FIGURE 4.10 T-Lymphoblastic lymphoma stained for CD3. The strong cytoplasmic positivity highlights nuclear clefts in this case.

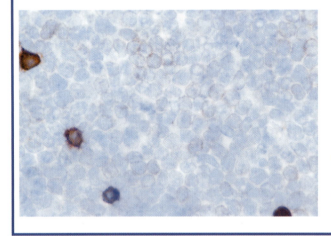

FIGURE 4.11 T-Lymphoblastic lymphoma stained for CD79a. In addition to the strong staining shown by three residual B-lymphocytes, some of the lymphoma cells show weak positivity.

MATURE B-CELL LYMPHOMAS

OVERVIEW

Mature B-cells are characterized by the synthesis, expression and sometimes secretion of immunoglobulin molecules. The almost infinite diversity of these molecules is achieved by rearrangement (shuffling) of the constant, joining, diversity and variable regions of the immunoglobulin genes. Further diversity occurs in follicle centres by the process of somatic mutation of the variable region genes. Thus, at the genetic level, mature B-cells are characterized by rearranged immunoglobulin genes. Follicle centre and postfollicle centre cells have mutated variable region genes.

Mature B-cell lymphomas will show clonal rearrangement of their immunoglobulin genes. Those that have arisen at the postfollicular stage of B-cell development will also show mutated variable region (v-region genes). Tumours arising at the follicle centre stage of B-cell maturation show ongoing mutations of the v-region genes (i.e. multiple mutations within a single clone). Analysis of the immunoglobulin genes provides a valuable means for the identification and subdivision of mature B-cell lymphomas.

B-cell lymphomas may be divided into those with a low growth fraction [chronic lymphocytic leukaemia/small lymphocytic lymphoma (CLL/SLL), lymphoplasmacytic lymphoma, mantle cell lymphoma, marginal zone lymphoma and follicular lymphoma] and high growth fraction lymphomas (diffuse large B-cell lymphoma and Burkitt lymphoma). A proportion of low growth fraction lymphomas transform into high growth fraction lymphomas. Low growth fraction lymphomas exhibit alterations in genes controlling apoptosis, whereas those with a high growth fraction have abnormalities of genes involving proliferation control (Sanchez-Beato *et al.* 2003).

There are reliable lineage-specific immunohistochemical markers for the identification of B-cells. The two most commonly used for paraffin-embedded tissues are CD20 and CD79a. Of these, CD79a is the most reliable, since it is expressed on cells from the pre-B-cell stage of maturation through to plasma cells. CD20 has a more limited range of expression, and may not be expressed on lymphomas representing the early and

Table 5.1: Common cytogenetic abnormalities found in mature B-cell lymphomas

LYMPHOMA	TRANSLOCATION	GENES INVOLVED
Lymphoplasmacytic lymphoma	t(9;14)(p13;q32)	PAX-5, IgH
Follicular lymphoma	t(14;18)(q32;q21)	IgH, BCL-2
Mantle cell lymphoma	t(11;14)(q13;q32)	BCL-1, IgH
Diffuse large B-cell lymphoma		
Approximately 30%	t(14;18)(q32;q21)	IgH, BCL-2
Approximately 30%	t(3;14)(q27;q32)	BCL-6, IgH
Very rare	t(2;17)(p23;q23)	ALK, clathrin
Burkitt lymphoma		
Approximately 80%	t(8;14)(q24;q32)	C-MYC, IgH
Approximately 10%	t(2;8)(q11;q24)	κ-light chain, C-MYC
Approximately 10%	t(8;22)(q24;q11)	C-MYC, λ-light chain

ALk, anaplastic lymphoma kinase; Ig, immunoglobulin.

late stages of B-cell differentiation. In addition to these lineage-specific markers, there are a number of antigens that are useful in identifying subtypes of B-cell lymphoma. These include CD5 (expressed on B-CLL/SLL and mantle cell lymphomas), CD10 (expressed on follicle centre cell lymphomas, B-lymphoblastic lymphoma and Burkitt lymphoma) and CD23 (expressed on B-CLL/SLL). The transcription factor bcl-6 is expressed in the nuclei of follicle centre cell-derived lymphomas.

The majority of mature B-cell lymphomas show characteristic chromosomal abnormalities, often translocations involving the immunoglobulin genes. These may provide markers for the various subtypes of B-cell lymphoma (Table 5.1). They may be identified by conventional cytogenetics, fluorescent *in-situ* hybridization (FISH) or by the polymerase chain reaction (PCR). A gene product overexpressed as a result of the translocation may be detectable by immunohistochemistry and provide a marker for the translocation, for example, cyclin D1 overexpressed in mantle cell lymphomas as a result of t(11;14).

Gene expression profiling of lymphomas is providing useful information that can identify different subgroups of lymphomas within a single diagnostic category. Thus, a study of small lymphocytic lymphomas was able to categorize borderline cases between B-CLL/SLL, mantle cell lymphoma and splenic marginal zone lymphoma (Thieblemont *et al.* 2004). Gene expression profiles of diffuse large B-cell lymphomas have identified good prognostic subtypes with expression profiles of germinal centre B-cells and poor prognosis subtypes with expression profiles of activated B-cells (Alizadeh *et al.* 2000). Gene expression profiling is an expensive and technically sophisticated process that requires the availability of unfixed tissue. Fortunately, the technique may identify genes of discriminatory value that may then be identified in fixed tissues using immunohistochemical techniques (Chang *et al.* 2004, Thieblemont *et al.* 2004).

These techniques, together with clinical features and morphology, have provided reliable methods for the identification and subclassification of mature B-cell lymphomas. This group of tumours comprises approximately 90 per cent of malignant lymphomas seen in most parts of the world. Diffuse large B-cell lymphoma is the commonest subtype, accounting for 30–40 per cent of all cases. In the developed world, follicular lymphomas account for over 20 per cent of cases.

B-CELL CHRONIC LYMPHOCYTIC LEUKAEMIA/SMALL LYMPHOCYTIC LYMPHOMA

Small lymphocytic lymphoma is usually regarded as the tissue manifestation of B-cell chronic lymphocytic leukaemia (B-CLL). Patients diagnosed as having B-CLL on blood and bone marrow examination often have some degree of lymphadenopathy. If lymph nodes from such patients are biopsied, they show the features of SLL, being diffusely infiltrated by small lymphocytes with scattered prolymphocytes and paraimmunoblasts. Some patients present with prominent lymphadenopathy and a lymph node biopsy may be the diagnostic procedure. In this 'tumour-forming' variant of B-CLL, the paraimmunoblasts are often aggregated into clusters, forming so-called proliferation centres. Most patients with 'tumour-forming' B-CLL will have, or will subsequently develop, the blood and bone marrow manifestations of this disease. A recent study of cases of B-CLL/SLL with and without prominent proliferation centres found no difference between these groups with respect to clinical features and immunophenotype (Asplund *et al.* 2002). In many cases of B-CLL/SLL, there is some preservation of the underlying nodal structure. Reticulin stains will often show preservation of sinus structures and residual reactive follicles may be seen.

Occasional cells in B-CLL/SLL may show immunoglobulin (Ig) inclusions, often appearing to be intranuclear (Dutcher bodies). These eosinophilic inclusions are usually of the IgM isotype and stain strongly with periodic acid–Schiff (PAS). In rare cases, a substantial number of the cells contain inclusions. Such cases were designated as lymphoplasmacytoid lymphomas in the Kiel classification. In all other respects, however, these cases have the morphology and immunophenotype of B-lymphocytic lymphoma and they should be regarded as a variant of this disease.

In rare cases of small lymphocytic lymphoma, paraimmunoblasts may form the predominant cell type. This has been referred to as the paraimmunoblastic variant of small lymphocytic lymphoma. It should not be confused with B-prolymphocytic leukaemia, which is clinically and phenotypically a different disease. Few cases of the paraimmunoblastic variant of small lymphocytic lymphoma have been studied and it is not known whether the prognosis of such cases is different from that of the more usual form of small lymphocytic lymphoma.

Another rare progression of small lymphocytic lymphoma is transformation to a diffuse large B-cell lymphoma, often referred to as Richter syndrome. Richter syndrome carries a poor prognosis. In very rare cases, a histological appearance indistinguishable from Hodgkin lymphoma develops. The tumour cells lose their B-cell markers and acquire the phenotype of Reed–Sternberg cells with a background infiltrate characteristic of Hodgkin lymphoma or of small lymphocytic lymphoma.

IMMUNOHISTOCHEMISTRY

B-Cell chronic lymphocytic leukaemia/SLL cells usually show weak expression of surface immunoglobulins

by flow cytometry. However, clear expression of perinuclear IgM and sometimes IgD together with light chains can usually be identified using immunohistochemistry. The B-cell associated antigens CD20 and CD79a are expressed, although CD79b and CD22 are usually weak or negative. The tumour cells are negative for CD10, but express CD5, CD23 and CD43. CD23 is fixation sensitive and often most strongly expressed on paraimmunoblasts. It is useful in the separation of B-lymphocytic lymphoma from mantle cell lymphoma. ZAP-70 the product of the *ZAP-70* gene can be demonstrated by flow cytometry and immunohistochemistry in cases of B-CLL/SLL with unmutated immunoglobulin genes (see later).

GENETICS

Most genetic studies of B-CLL have been performed on blood and marrow with few studies of tissue infiltrates. The disease appears to be heterogeneous. Trisomy 12 is found in 10–15 per cent of cases by cytogenetics and in 20 per cent of cases using interphase FISH. Only a proportion of the clone, identified by the Ig phenotype, exhibits trisomy 12, suggesting that this is probably a secondary genetic event. Twenty per cent of B-CLLs show deletions of chromosome 13q14 by routine cytogenetics and 60 per cent show this deletion by interphase FISH. Deletions of chromosome 11q13 are found in less than 5 per cent of patients cytogenetically but in 20 per cent using interphase FISH. Mutations of the gene for p53 occur in 10–15 per cent of cases.

Rearranged immunoglobulin heavy and light chain genes are found in B-CLL. Mutational patterns in the variable region genes of over half the cases suggest that these cases have been exposed to the mutational influence of the germinal centre. Cases with mutated Ig genes are more likely to be Binet stage A with stable disease, typical lymphocyte morphology and to have deletions of 13q14. Cases lacking mutations (naive cells) are associated with progressive disease, atypical morphology and trisomy 12. Gene expression profiling has shown that *ZAP-70* (expressed in unmutated cases) is the gene that best distinguishes these two prognostic subtypes (Weistner *et al.* 2003).

DIFFERENTIAL DIAGNOSIS

The main differential diagnosis of SLL is with mantle cell lymphoma. In the latter, the cells are usually more angulated than small lymphocytes but may appear rounded. The presence of paraimmunoblasts, either singly or in clusters, identifies small lymphocytic lymphoma. On fresh or optimally fixed tissues the detection of CD23 identifies SLL. Nuclear expression of cyclin D1 identifies mantle cell lymphomas. Cases of SLL with prominent proliferation centres may be mistaken for follicle centre cell lymphoma (FCCL). Small lymphocytic lymphoma shows some preservation of the underlying reticulin structure of the node and does not show the nodular reticulin pattern characteristic of FCCL. The paraimmunoblasts in proliferation centres have more delicate nuclear chromatin and a more uniform nuclear size than the centroblasts of FCCL. Immunohistochemistry will differentiate B-CLL/SLL (CD5+, CD23+) from FCCL (CD10+, bcl-6+).

▲ BOX 5.1: B-Cell chronic lymphocytic leukaemia/small lymphocytic lymphoma: clinical features

- ▲ Median age 65 years
- ▲ Male predominance 2:1
- ▲ Most patients have bone marrow involvement (stage IV)
- ▲ Presenting features
  Asymptomatic (incidental finding)
  Fatigue
  Autoimmune haemolytic anaemia
  Infections
  Splenomegaly
  Lymphadenopathy

● BOX 5.2: B-Cell chronic lymphocytic leukaemia/small lymphocytic lymphoma: morphology

- Architecture of node partially preserved
- Diffuse infiltrate of lymphocytes with clumped chromatin
- Prolymphocytes or paraimmunoblasts, either singly or forming 'proliferation centres'
- Immunoglobulin inclusions (uncommon)
- Transformation (rare)
  Diffuse large B-cell lymphoma (Richter syndrome)
  Hodgkin lymphoma

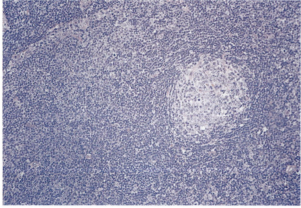

FIGURE 5.1 B-Cell chronic lymphocytic leukaemia/small lymphocytic lymphoma. Low-power view showing residual germinal centre surrounded by tumour cells.

FIGURE 5.2 B-Cell chronic lymphocytic leukaemia/small lymphocytic lymphoma. Low-power view showing pale proliferation centres.

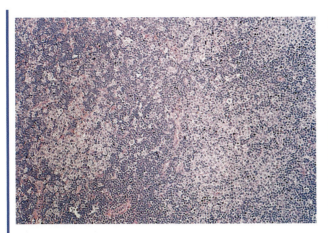

FIGURE 5.3 B-Cell chronic lymphocytic leukaemia/small lymphocytic lymphoma showing proliferation centres containing many paraimmunoblasts.

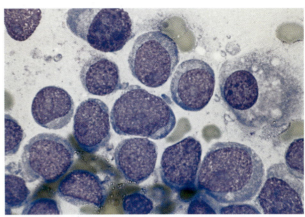

FIGURE 5.4 B-Cell chronic lymphocytic leukaemia/small lymphocytic lymphoma. Paraimmunoblastic variant imprint preparation showing fine chromatin, visible nucleoli and cytoplasmic basophilia.

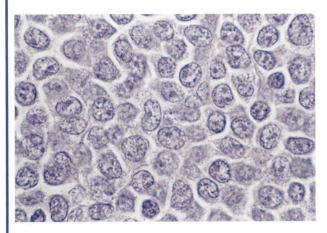

FIGURE 5.5 B-Cell chronic lymphocytic leukaemia/small lymphocytic lymphoma paraimmunoblastic variant in which most of the cells resemble paraimmunoblasts.

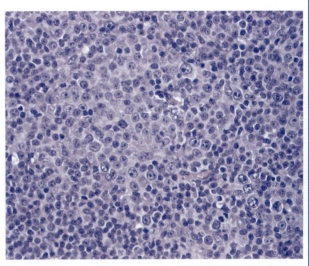

FIGURE 5.6 Proliferation centre showing paraimmunoblasts with small lymphocytes at the periphery.

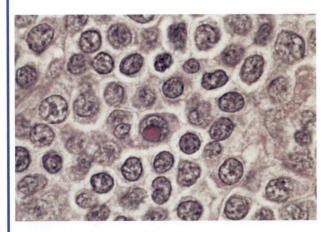

FIGURE 5.7 B-Cell chronic lymphocytic leukaemia/small lymphocytic lymphoma. Periodic acid Schiff stain showing intranuclear inclusion of immunoglobulin M (IgM; Dutcher body).

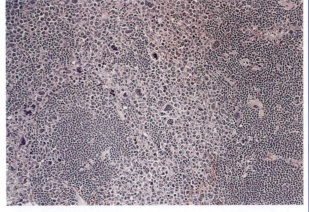

FIGURE 5.8 B-Cell chronic lymphocytic leukaemia/small lymphocytic lymphoma showing transformation to high-grade lymphoma (Richter syndrome).

◆ **BOX 5.3: B-Cell chronic lymphocytic leukaemia/small lymphocytic lymphoma: immunohistochemistry**

- ◆ IgM together with light chain detectable in many cases
- ◆ IgD may be detected
- ◆ CD20+
- ◆ CD79a+

- ◆ CD5+
- ◆ CD23+
- ◆ ZAP-70+ in most cases with unmutated immunoglobulin genes

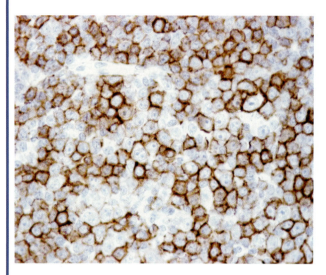

FIGURE 5.9 Membrane staining of B-cells for CD23. Strongest staining seen on paraimmunoblasts.

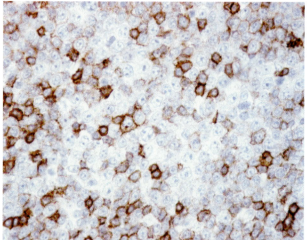

FIGURE 5.10 Proliferation centre showing strong CD5 positivity of small T-lymphocytes with variable membrane staining of paraimmunoblasts.

B-CELL PROLYMPHOCYTIC LEUKAEMIA

B-cell prolymphocytic leukaemia (B-PLL) is a rare B-cell neoplasm in patients with a mean age of 70 years and has a male predominance of 1.6:1. Patients usually present with marked splenomegaly and a high white cell count; lymphadenopathy is uncommon. In tissue sections, the tumour cells are approximately twice the size of lymphocytes. The nuclei are generally rounded with finely granular chromatin and a single prominent central nucleolus. When lymph nodes are involved they show a diffuse or vaguely nodular infiltration.

B-cell prolymphocytic leukaemia cells express surface IgM with or without IgD. The B-cell antigens CD20 and CD79a are positive. CD5 is expressed in approximately one-third of the cases and CD23 is usually negative.

Approximately 20 per cent of cases of B-PLL have been reported to show t(11;14)(q13;q32), but it may

be that these are examples of the blastoid variant of mantle cell lymphoma.

DIFFERENTIAL DIAGNOSIS

B-cell prolymphocytic leukaemia is not the same as B-CLL, with large numbers of prolymphocytes and paraimmunoblasts (paraimmunoblastic variant of B-CLL). These two diseases can usually be distinguished by their clinical and immunophenotypic features. Cases showing t(11;14) and expressing cyclin D1 are likely to be blastoid variants of mantle cell lymphoma rather than B-PLL. The exact relationship between B-PLL and hairy cell leukaemia variant (prolymphocytoid variant) is uncertain.

LYMPHOPLASMACYTIC LYMPHOMA/IMMUNOCYTOMA

A number of B-cell lymphomas may show plasma cell differentiation. This is a common and characteristic feature of both nodal and extranodal marginal zone lymphomas. It is rarely seen in follicle centre cell lymphomas and is not seen in mantle cell lymphomas. Such cases showing plasma cell differentiation may in the past have been categorized as lymphoplasmacytic lymphomas. The term immunocytomas lymphoplasmacytoid type was used in the Kiel classification for lymphocytic tumours containing large numbers of immunoglobulin inclusions. These tumours, which are CD5 and CD23+, are now regarded as a variant of B-CLL/SLL. Thus, the diagnosis of lymphoplasmacytic lymphoma should be made only in the absence of features of other B-cell lymphomas, such as neoplastic follicles or monocytoid B-cells.

Lymphoplasmacytic lymphoma is a clonal proliferation of small lymphocytes and plasma cells with intermediate plasmacytoid forms. Patients most commonly present with bone marrow and splenic disease; presentation with lymphadenopathy is less common. Lymph nodes involved by lymphoplasmacytic lymphoma show a diffuse infiltrate of small lymphocytes, plasma cells and intermediate forms. These cells are best seen in Giemsa-stained preparations. The plasma cells are not uniformly distributed, but often aggregate adjacent to sinuses or fibrous trabeculae. Cytoplasmic and intranuclear inclusions of immunoglobulin (Dutcher bodies) are often present in a proportion of the plasma cells and are highlighted by PAS staining.

Many lymphoplasmacytic lymphomas show preservation of the underlying nodal architecture and frequently exhibit marked dilatation of the sinuses often associated with haemosiderosis. The dilated sinuses are filled with eosinophilic proteinaceous fluid as well as tumour cells. Scattered mast cells are a characteristic feature of lymphoplasmacytic lymphoma infiltrates at all sites. Variable numbers of epithelioid histiocytes may be present. Andriko et al. (2001) described three histological patterns among 20 cases of lymphoplasmacytic lymphoma. Seven cases had the histological pattern described above, four showed hyperplastic follicles and nine showed diffuse effacement of the nodal structure with variable fibrosis. Amyloid was present in two cases.

Some cases of lymphoplasmacytic lymphoma are associated with Waldenstrom macroglobulinaemia. Waldenstrom macroglobulinaemia should not, however, be regarded as a specific histological diagnosis, since it is also rarely associated with splenic marginal zone lymphoma, B-CLL and extranodal marginal zone lymphoma.

Lymphoplasmacytic lymphomas often contain variable numbers of immunoblasts and may show progression to a diffuse large B-cell lymphoma of immunoblastic type (immunoblastic lymphoma).

IMMUNOHISTOCHEMISTRY

The tumour cells express surface and cytoplasmic immunoglobulin of the IgM isotype, and less commonly of the IgG isotype, showing light chain restriction. They express the B-cell markers CD20 and CD79a, but are negative for CD5 and CD10. It should be noted that CD20 is often not expressed on the plasma cell component of the tumour. The plasma cell markers CD38 and CD138 are usually positive.

GENETICS

The immunoglobulin genes are rearranged and mutated, as in postgerminal centre cells. Some lymphoplasmacytic lymphomas have been shown to have the t(9;14)(p13;q32) chromosomal translocation. This translocation juxtaposes the PAX-5 gene at 9q13 with the regulatory elements of the immunoglobulin heavy

---

▲ BOX 5.4: Lymphoplasmacytic lymphoma/immunocytoma: clinical features

- ▲ Median age 63 years
- ▲ Slight male predominance
- ▲ Sites of involvement
  Bone marrow
  Blood
  Spleen
  Lymph nodes
- ▲ Most patients have monoclonal immunoglobulin M (IgM) paraprotein (Waldenstrom's macroglobulinaemia). May have hyperviscosity syndrome, neuropathy, IgM deposits in skin and gastrointestinal tract
- ▲ Cases expressing IgG or more rarely IgA do not have hyperviscosity syndrome
- ▲ Reported association with hepatitis C infection

● BOX 5.5: Lymphoplasmacytic lymphoma/immunocytoma: morphology

- Nodal architecture often partially preserved
- Infiltrate composed of small lymphocytes, plasma cells and intermediate lymphoplasmacytoid forms
- Intranuclear IgM inclusions (Dutcher bodies)
- Sinuses dilated and filled with eosinophilic proteinaceous material

- Haemosiderosis
- Variable fibrosis
- Amyloid deposition (uncommon)
- Increased numbers of mast cells

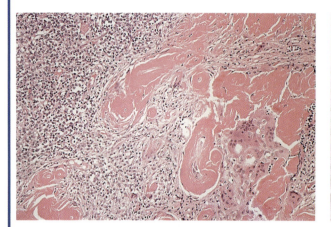

FIGURE 5.11 Lymphoplasmacytic lymphoma showing amyloid deposition. Note the giant cell reaction to the amyloid.

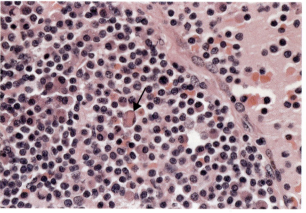

FIGURE 5.12 Lymphoplasmacytic lymphoma showing dilated sinus containing pink proteinaceous material. The adjacent cells are lymphocytes and plasma cells. The arrow indicates a Dutcher body.

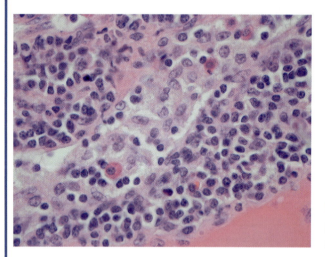

FIGURE 5.13 High-power view of lymphoplasmacytic lymphoma showing parasinusoidal distribution of lymphocytes and plasma cells. Three mast cells are present in the sinus.

◆ BOX 5.6: Lymphoplasmacytic lymphoma/immunocytoma: immunohistochemistry

- Cytoplasmic IgM+, expression of immunoglobulin G (IgG) and IgA less common
- Cytoplasmic/intranuclear IgM inclusions
- CD20+, but often negative on plasma cells

- CD79a+
- CD5, CD10, CD23−
- CD38 and CD138+ on plasma cells

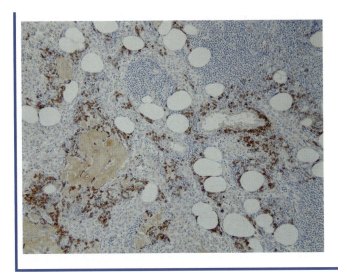

FIGURE 5.14 Lymphoplasmacytic lymphoma showing strong κ positivity of plasma cells that accumulate around vessels and fibrous trabeculae.

chain gene at 14q32, leading to deregulation of the PAX-5 gene. The PAX-5 gene encodes a B-cell specific transcription factor.

DIFFERENTIAL DIAGNOSIS

Differentiation from reactive lymphadenopathy with many plasma cells (e.g. as in rheumatoid disease) can usually be made on the basis of the more obvious reactive features in the latter. The identification of light chain restriction in lymphoplasmacytic lymphoma confirms the neoplastic nature of the infiltrate. Other B-cell lymphomas showing plasma cell differentiation, such as marginal zone lymphomas, can usually be differentiated from lymphoplasmacytic lymphomas by the presence of other characteristic cell types, such as monocytoid B-cells. In some cases, amyloidosis may be so extensive that the appearances suggest primary amyloidosis. In such cases, a careful search should be made for residual islands of lymphoplasmacytic lymphoma.

HAIRY CELL LEUKAEMIA

Hairy cell leukaemia is an uncommon B-cell neoplasm that primarily involves the bone marrow, blood and spleen. The name is derived from the appearance of the lymphoid cells in peripheral blood smears, where they show hairy cytoplasmic projections. The disease has a median age of 55 years and a male to female ratio of 5:1. Patients most commonly present with pancytopaenia and splenomegaly. Lymph node involvement in hairy cell leukaemia is rare, although lymphadenopathy caused by intercurrent opportunistic infections, as a consequence of the immunodeficiency associated with this disease, may occur. When lymph nodes are involved by hairy cell leukaemia, the infiltrate is diffuse, involving the paracortex and eventually the whole node.

The cells of hairy cell leukaemia are about twice the size of small lymphocytes. Their nuclear chromatin is less heterochromatic than that of B-CLL cells. In tissue sections, their nuclei are usually oval or bean shaped, and are surrounded by an ill-defined zone of clear cytoplasm ('fried-egg' appearance). Obstruction of the microcirculation may lead to blood lakes and pseudoangiomatous formations.

IMMUNOHISTOCHEMISTRY

The tumour cells express surface immunoglobulin and B-cell associated antigens. They are usually negative for CD5, CD10 and CD23. They strongly express CD11c and CD25, but these are not specific. CD103, which also labels epitheliotropic mucosal T-cells, is more specific but not applicable to fixed tissue sections. The monoclonal antibody DBA44 labels these cells in fixed tissue sections, but is not entirely specific.

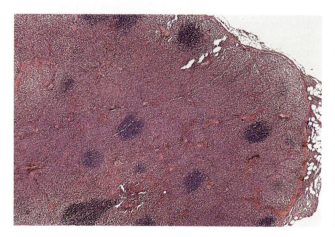

FIGURE 5.15 Hairy cell leukaemia. Splenic hilar lymph node showing residual follicles pushed apart by pale-staining hairy cells.

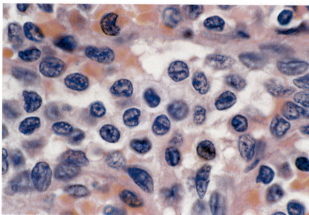

FIGURE 5.16 Hairy cell leukaemia. High-power view showing the grooved bean-shaped nuclei of the hairy cells and their abundant pale cytoplasm.

GENETICS

The immunoglobulin heavy and light chain genes are rearranged and mutated. Cyclin D1 is overexpressed in over half the cases of hairy cell leukaemia, but this is not associated with translocation of the BCL-1 gene.

PLASMACYTOMA

Most pathologists will be familiar with bone marrow-derived plasma cell tumours presenting as single or multiple osteolytic tumours (multiple myeloma). Soft tissue plasmacytomas do not appear to be related to multiple myelomatosis. They occur most frequently in the upper aerodigestive tract. Primary plasmacytoma of the lymph nodes is uncommon and metastasis from a soft tissue plasmacytoma should be excluded before making this diagnosis.

Lymph nodes may be completely or partially replaced by the neoplastic infiltrate. The tumour cells may have the typical cytological appearances of mature plasma cells. The plasmablastic form has a more blastic morphology with an open chromatin structure and visible nucleoli. Anaplastic plasmacytomas may show considerable morphological variability and need to be differentiated from large cell lymphomas and other anaplastic neoplasms. Tumour cells may contain immunoglobulin inclusions in the form of globules or, more rarely, crystalloids. Extracellular eosinophilic material is commonly seen and it may form the most prominent histological feature. In some cases, but not all, this material is amyloid giving positive staining with Congo red stain and showing characteristic anomalous colours in polarized light. Amyloid frequently elicits a foreign-body giant cell reaction.

IMMUNOHISTOCHEMISTRY

Plasma cells lose many of the surface markers that characterize mature B-cells. Thus, they are frequently negative for CD45, and CD20, but usually do express CD79a. The tumour cells synthesize immunoglobulin, most commonly of the IgA or IgG isotype, and show light-chain restriction. A number of antibodies, relatively specific for plasma cells, such as CD38 and CD138, may be of diagnostic value. Normal and neoplastic plasma cells commonly express epithelial membrane antigen (EMA), and rare cases may express cytoplasmic cytokeratin.

GENETICS

There are numerous cytogenetic studies of myeloma. It is uncertain how these relate to soft tissue or, more specifically, lymph node plasmacytomas. All cases

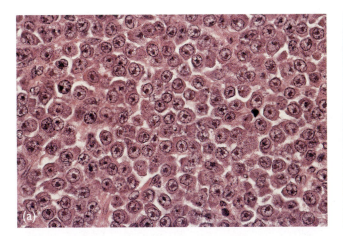

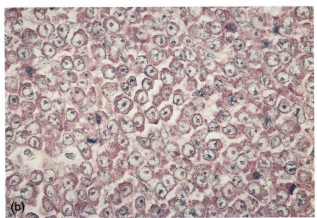

FIGURE 5.17 (a) Plasmacytoma, plasmablastic type showing prominent nucleoli and dark amphophilic cytoplasm. (b) Stained by methyl green pyronin to demonstrate cytoplasmic RNA.

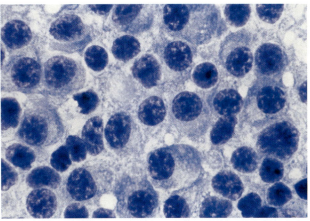

FIGURE 5.18 Imprint preparation of plasmacytoma showing the appearance of mature plasma cells.

of myeloma exhibit translocations involving the immunoglobulin genes. Some of these are recurrent, whereas others appear random and rare. Many involve the switch region of the immunoglobulin heavy chain gene, consistent with the expression of IgA or IgG by many of these tumours. The translocation t(11;14)(q13;q32) occurs in 20–25 per cent of myelomas, leading to overexpression of cyclin D1. This should be borne in mind when using antibodies to cyclin D1 to confirm the diagnosis of mantle cell lymphoma.

DIFFERENTIAL DIAGNOSIS

Intense plasma cell proliferation may occur in reactive and inflammatory lymphadenopathies. The plasma cells are typically well differentiated, with condensed nuclear chromatin and basophilic cytoplasm. They are most characteristically distributed in the medullary

cords of the lymph node. The association with other inflammatory cells and reactive features will usually distinguish these proliferations from plasmacytoma. The demonstration of light-chain restriction will usually make the distinction in difficult cases. Plasmacytoma and lymphoplasmacytic lymphoma should always be excluded in lymph nodes showing amyloidosis.

Castleman's disease of the plasmacytic subtype can usually be differentiated from plasmacytoma by the presence of characteristic hyalinized follicles. Some patients with this disease show λ-light chain restriction. Lymphoplasmacytic lymphoma rarely presents with lymphadenopathy. The presence of small lymphocytes, plasma cells and intermediate forms differentiates lymphoplasmacytic lymphoma from the more homogeneous plasma cell infiltrates of plasmacytoma.

Marginal zone lymphomas may show extreme plasma cell differentiation, leading to confusion with plasmacytoma. They can usually be differentiated by the presence of characteristic marginal zone cells and often by the presence of large numbers of epithelioid histiocytes.

The differentiation of blastic and anaplastic plasmacytomas from large cell lymphomas may be difficult, particularly those showing the characteristic morphology of immunoblastic lymphoma, with large single nucleoli and basophilic cytoplasm. The expression of CD45, and CD20 would favour the diagnosis of large B-cell lymphoma, whereas the absence of these markers and the presence of EMA and plasma cell antigens would favour plasmacytoma. The absence of leucocyte common antigen (CD45) and the presence of EMA and, very rarely, cytokeratin in an anaplastic plasmacytoma might lead the unwary into a diagnosis of anaplastic carcinoma or anaplastic large cell lymphoma.

NODAL MARGINAL ZONE LYMPHOMA (MONOCYTOID B-CELL LYMPHOMA)

Monocytoid B-cells were first described in lymphadenitis due to toxoplasmosis and other reactive lymphadenopathies. The cells were originally thought to be of the monocyte macrophage lineage and the appearance was referred to as immature sinus histiocytosis. After immunohistochemical analysis showed the cells to be B-cells, they were redesignated as monocytoid B-cells. It is often assumed that nodal marginal zone lymphomas are derived from monocytoid B-cells despite the fact that the two cell types show differences in their molecular and immunohistochemical characteristics (Camacho et al. 2003). Following the description of monocytoid B-cell lymphoma at nodal and extranodal sites, it became apparent that these tumours were morphologically and immunophenotypically similar to extranodal marginal zone (MALT) lymphoma. Analysis of several series of nodal monocytoid lymphomas showed an association with synchronous or metachronous extranodal marginal zone lymphoma in many, but not all, cases. It thus appears that the presence of a nodal monocytoid B-cell lymphoma is often a manifestation of an underlying overt or occult MALT lymphoma. It was subsequently shown that a small proportion of nodal marginal zone lymphomas have the immunophenotype of splenic marginal zone lymphoma rather than extranodal marginal zone lymphoma (splenic marginal zone lymphomas often express IgD and are CD43−, whereas extranodal marginal zone lymphomas are IgD− and often CD43+). These cases, however, did not have evidence of splenic disease at the time of lymph node biopsy (Campo et al. 1999).

The cells of nodal marginal zone B-cell lymphoma have small to medium-sized nuclei that are rounded indented or irregular. They have abundant pale or clear cytoplasm. It is this cytoplasmic pallor that makes clusters of monocytoid B-cells stand out in histological sections. The cells are often distributed within or alongside sinuses and are generally interfollicular. Colonization of the reactive follicles occurs as the disease progresses.

Tumours frequently show plasma cell differentiation, the plasma cells exhibiting the same monoclonal immunoglobulin within their cytoplasm as is found on the surface of the monocytoid B-cells. Epithelioid cell clusters are also commonly found in monocytoid B-cell lymphomas, particularly those associated with autoimmune sialadenitis. Epithelioid cells frequently surround small groups of monocytoid B-cells.

IMMUNOPHENOTYPE

Tumour cells express surface immunoglobulin, usually of the IgM class, sometimes in association with IgD; IgG or IgA are less commonly expressed. Cells showing plasma cell differentiation show cytoplasmic immunoglobulin of the same class and express plasma cell-associated antigens. The monocytoid cells express the B-cell-associated antigens CD20 and CD79a. They are usually negative for CD5, although rare CD5+ cases, usually with blood and bone marrow involvement, have been reported (Ballesteros et al. 1998). They do not express CD10 or CD23. Abnormal expression of apoptosis regulator proteins has been reported (Camacho et al. 2003).

GENETICS

Probably because of its rarity, the genotype of nodal marginal zone B-cell lymphoma is uncertain. Studies of extranodal marginal lymphomas have shown the translocation t(11;18)(q21;q21) in approximately one-third of low-grade cases. The genes involved are the apoptosis inhibitor gene AP12 and a novel gene MLT. Another non-random translocation, t(1;14)(p22;q32), occurs in less than 5 per cent of extranodal marginal lymphomas. This translocation involves the immunoglobulin heavy-chain gene on chromosome 14 and the BCL10 gene on chromosome 1. Suppression of apoptosis may be the consequence of both of these translocations. A number of trisomies have been

---

▲ **BOX 5.7: Nodal marginal zone lymphoma (monocytoid B-cell lymphoma): clinical features**

- ▲ Less than 2 per cent of all non-Hodgkin lymphomas
- ▲ 30–50 per cent have associated extranodal marginal zone lymphomas
- ▲ Rare cases associated with splenic marginal zone lymphoma
- ▲ Sites of involvement:
    Peripheral lymph nodes, localized or generalized
    Bone marrow
    Peripheral blood

● BOX 5.8: Nodal marginal zone lymphoma (monocytoid B-cell lymphoma): morphology

- Partial preservation of nodal architecture
- Marginal zone B-cells infiltrate interfollicular areas, within or adjacent to sinuses
- Follicular colonization
- Nuclei rounded, oval or cleaved
- Clear cytoplasm
- Plasma cell differentiation in some cases
- Infiltrate of epithelioid histiocytes in some cases
- Scattered blast cells
- May transform to large B-cell lymphoma

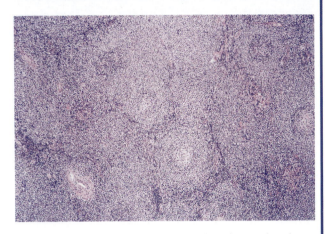

FIGURE 5.21 Nodal marginal zone lymphoma showing nodular growth pattern with reactive follicles at the centre of the nodules. Note the paler staining marginal zone cells around the follicles.

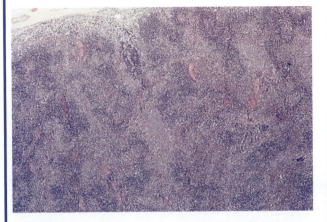

FIGURE 5.19 Nodal marginal zone lymphoma. The pale marginal zone cells follow the distribution of the lymph node sinuses.

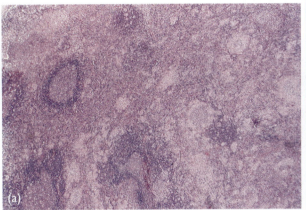

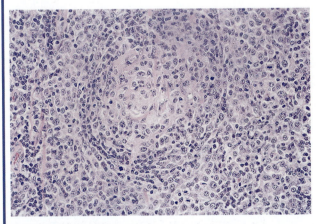

FIGURE 5.20 Higher power view of nodal marginal zone lymphoma showing a reactive germinal centre surrounded by an attenuated mantle zone of small lymphocytes with an outer zone of marginal zone cells.

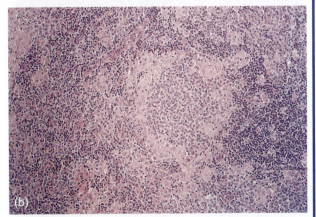

FIGURE 5.22 (a, b) Nodal marginal zone lymphoma. Showing residual reactive follicles and islands of marginal zone cells surrounded by epithelioid histiocytes.

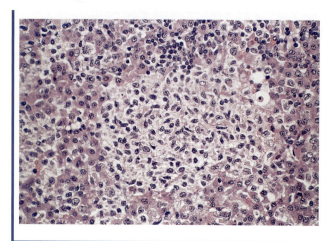

FIGURE 5.23 Nodal marginal zone lymphoma showing plasmacytic differentiation.

◆ **BOX 5.9: Nodal marginal zone lymphoma (monocytoid B-cell lymphoma): immunohistochemistry**

- Surface/cytoplasmic IgM or, less commonly, IgA or IgG
- IgD − except in splenic marginal zone type
- CD20 and CD79a+
- CD5 usually negative

- CD10 and CD23−
- CD43 usually positive except in splenic marginal zone type
- Tumour cells bcl-2+; residual reactive follicles bcl-2−.

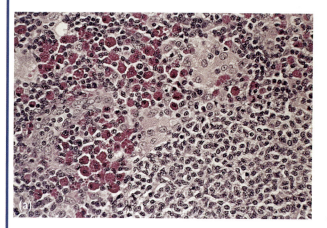
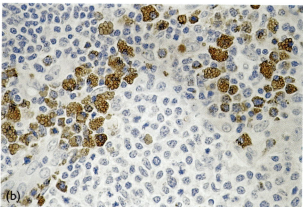

FIGURE 5.24 Nodal marginal zone lymphoma with plasmacytic differentiation. (a) Periodic acid Schiff stain showing inclusions of immunoglobulin M (IgM) within the plasma cells. (b) Same case stained for IgM.

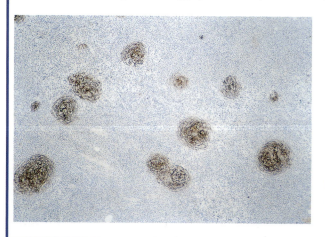

FIGURE 5.25 Low-power view of nodal marginal zone lymphoma stained for CD21, showing residual follicular dendritic cells.

reported in MALT lymphomas; however, these are usually associated with complex karyotypes and may, therefore, be secondary events. Immunoglobulin genes are mutated in most cases.

DIFFERENTIAL DIAGNOSIS

Nodal monocytoid B-cell lymphoma must be separated from reactive lymphadenopathies associated with monocytoid B-cell hyperplasia. These include toxoplasmic lymphadenitis and human immunodeficiency virus (HIV)-associated lymphadenitis. In the original descriptions of nodal monocytoid B-cell lymphoma,

it was stated that demonstration of immunoglobulin light-chain restriction might be necessary to make this distinction (Sheibani *et al.* 1986, 1988). The presence of characteristic monocytoid cells distinguishes this lymphoma from lymphoplasmacytic lymphoma. The presence of numerous epithelioid cells is characteristic of many monocytoid B-cell lymphomas but less common in lymphoplasmacytic lymphoma. Rare follicular lymphomas showing marginal zone differentiation may mimic nodal marginal zone B-cell lymphoma. In these tumours, the follicles have the characteristics of neoplastic follicles, including bcl-2 positivity, in contrast to the reactive follicles present in nodal marginal zone B-cell lymphoma.

FOLLICULAR LYMPHOMA

Follicular lymphomas are the commonest subtype of low-grade non-Hodgkin lymphoma in the Western world, being most prevalent in the USA. They are less common in Africa and Asia. The tumour is rare in childhood and has its maximum incidence in the sixth and seventh decades of life. Follicular lymphoma usually presents with lymphadenopathy. Involvement of the bone marrow and the spleen is common and most patients present with stage III or stage IV disease. Patients with bone marrow involvement may show overspill of lymphoma cells into the peripheral blood. Involvement of extranodal sites, such as the tonsil, intestine and skin, is relatively uncommon. The disease usually runs a progressive course, though even without therapy, it may undergo spontaneous remission for varying lengths of time. Chemotherapy may be used to control the disease but it is rarely curative.

HISTOLOGY

The follicles of follicular lymphoma are usually closely packed, extend throughout the node and have relatively uniform rounded outlines. They may extend into and replace the fat in the hilum of the node, frequently seen in axillary lymph nodes, and they also extend into the perinodal fat. The pre-existing nodal architecture is distorted and destroyed with loss of the sinus structure.

Follicular lymphomas are derived from follicle centre B-cells and are composed of variable mixtures of centroblasts and centrocytes. The neoplastic follicles, like their reactive counterparts contain dendritic reticulum

cells and reactive T-cells, mainly of the CD4 subset. Neoplastic follicles often acquire a mantle of non-neoplastic small B-cells, though this is usually more attenuated and less well defined than that of reactive follicles. There is a tendency for follicular lymphomas to become more blastic (acquire a larger proportion of centroblasts) with time, a trend that is often associated with the acquisition of further cytogenetic abnormalities. The trend towards a more blastic morphology is also associated with the development of areas of diffuse growth, so that the tumour may become follicular and diffuse or completely diffuse.

The predominant interfollicular cells in many follicular lymphomas are small B- or T-cells. However, tumour cells are often found in this situation, recognizable by their morphology or by their immunohistochemical staining.

In their cytomorphology, the tumour cells of many follicular lymphomas resemble normal centroblasts or centrocytes. The tumour cells in other cases, particularly of the higher grades, may show an atypical morphology. Centroblasts may show multilobated, serpiginous or multinucleated nuclei. Centrocytes may also show dysplastic changes.

GRADING OF FOLLICULAR LYMPHOMAS

In 1982, Mann and Berard proposed a method for the cytological subclassification (grading) of follicular lymphomas. This system is based on the number of centroblasts per high power field, with 0–5 being grade 1, 6–15 grade 2, and 16 or more grade 3. The prognostic value of the Mann and Berard grading system has been widely studied and debated and, despite its shortcomings, its use has been recommended in the World Health Organisation (WHO) classification. Grading may influence patient management, for example, patients with grade 1 tumours may not be treated, or be offered only symptomatic treatment, whereas grade 3 tumours will usually be treated with chemotherapy. Patients with grade 3 follicular lymphoma have earlier relapses than grades 1 and 2, but similar overall survival. The poorer freedom from relapse of grade 3 disease may be overridden by chemotherapy.

The ability to recognize blasts depends on the fixation, thickness and quality of the section. Giemsa-stained sections in which the basophilia of the centroblast cytoplasm highlights these cells may be helpful. The grade is determined by counting ten fields and taking the average, since the grade may vary between follicles.

Follicular lymphomas may have areas of diffuse growth pattern and both the REAL and the WHO Classifications recommend that the degree of follicularity should be reported as follows:

1. predominantly follicular – >75 per cent follicular;
2. follicular and diffuse – 25–75 per cent follicular;
3. predominantly diffuse – <25 per cent follicular.

The significance of this subclassification with respect to treatment or survival is uncertain.

In grade 3 tumours, diffuse areas represent areas of diffuse large B-cell lymphoma. Such cases should not be reported as follicular and diffuse, but as follicular lymphoma grade 3 (x per cent) with diffuse large B-cell lymphoma (y per cent). The presence of diffuse large B-cell lymphoma usually dictates more aggressive therapy.

Grade 3 follicular lymphomas should be further subdivided into those with residual centrocytes (3A) and those without centrocytes (3B). A recent study of follicular lymphoma grade 3B has shown that cases can be separated into those with t(14;18) involving the BCL-2 gene, those with 3q27 abnormalities involving the BCL-6 gene, and those with neither of these but with other cytogenetic aberrations. Those with t(14;18) are probably related to the spectrum of follicular lymphomas, whereas those with 3q27 or other aberrations are more closely related to the majority of diffuse large B-cell lymphomas (Bosga–Bower et al. 2003).

MORPHOLOGICAL VARIATION WITHIN FOLLICULAR LYMPHOMAS

Within the category of follicular lymphomas, there is considerable variation in histological appearances.

Depending on the number of centroblasts and centrocytes in, and between, the follicles and the prominence, or otherwise, of the mantle zone, the follicles may be well defined or barely discernible. Follicularity may be highlighted by reticulin staining and is often accentuated by immunohistochemical staining for B- and T-cells. Other morphological variations are as given below.

SCLEROSIS

Sclerosis is a common feature of follicular lymphomas, particularly those involving the retroperitoneal lymph nodes. It frequently takes the form of fine or coarse fibrous bands surrounding groups of neoplastic follicles. Sometimes it surrounds and partially obliterates individual follicles. Less commonly, it is seen within follicles. Sclerosis has no prognostic significance.

AMORPHOUS, PAS-POSITIVE, EXTRACELLULAR MATERIAL

Eosinophilic amorphous material may be found in reactive and in neoplastic follicles, where it may be so abundant that it obscures the tumour cells. Unlike collagen, this material is non-birefringent. Electron microscopic examination shows it to be composed of membranous material.

IMMUNOGLOBULIN INCLUSIONS

Immunoglobulin, most frequently of the IgM isotype, may accumulate in the endoplasmic reticulum or perinuclear space. In the former, it appears as Russell bodies and, in the latter, as intranuclear inclusions. The inclusions are usually strongly PAS positive.

SIGNET RING LYMPHOMA

Clear cytoplasmic inclusions that displace and compress the nucleus may be seen in a few or many tumour cells of a follicular lymphoma. These vacuoles do not stain with PAS. They have been reported to contain monoclonal IgG but it is often not possible to demonstrate immunoglobulin in these cases. Ultrastructurally, the vacuoles are seen to contain membranes and vesicles.

FOLLICULAR LYMPHOMA WITH PLASMACYTIC DIFFERENTIATION

A small number of follicle centre cell lymphomas show plasma cell differentiation with either intrafollicular or interfollicular monoclonal plasma cells.

FOLLICULAR LYMPHOMA WITH ATYPICAL NUCLEAR MORPHOLOGY

Rarely, follicular lymphomas show cells with cerebriform nuclei similar to those seen in the tumour cells of mycosis fungoides. The centroblasts within follicular lymphomas may show multilobated or serpiginous (centrocytoid) nuclei.

FLORAL VARIANT OF FOLLICULAR LYMPHOMA

In this uncommon variant of follicular lymphoma, the neoplastic follicle centres are broken up by ingrowths of small lymphocytes, giving an irregular flower-like outline to the follicles. The importance of recognizing this subtype is that it may be mistaken for progressive transformation of germinal centres or for nodular lymphocyte-predominant Hodgkin lymphoma.

FOLLICULAR LYMPHOMA WITH MONOCYTOID B-CELL DIFFERENTIATION

Monocytoid B-cell differentiation in follicular lymphomas is more commonly seen in the spleen than in lymph nodes. Pale-staining collars of cells surround the neoplastic follicles. These cells are part of the neoplastic clone that has acquired more abundant clear or pale-staining cytoplasm. These cases may mimic monocytoid B-cell lymphoma morphologically. In monocytoid B-cell lymphoma the follicles are reactive and, therefore, will be bcl-2− and will not show light-chain restriction.

FOLLICULAR LYMPHOMA WITH TOTAL INFARCTION OF LYMPH NODE

Infarction of lymph nodes usually occurs in lymph nodes involved by lymphoma and, most commonly, in those involved by follicular lymphoma. Multiple blocks should be examined to look for residual non-infarcted tissue. Reticulin staining may reveal underlying structural details that are not apparent in haematoxylin and eosin (H&E) or Giemsa-stained sections. Some antigens, detectable by immunohistochemistry, survive for a considerable time following infarction allowing the distribution and the phenotype of the tumour cells to be determined.

COMPOSITE LYMPHOMA

Follicular lymphomas may show areas of higher grade or diffuse growth pattern. These are not composite lymphomas but lymphomas showing tumour progression.

Hodgkin lymphoma occasionally develops within a low-grade lymphoma; most commonly follicular lymphoma. In these cases, the Hodgkin lymphoma has the morphology and phenotype of one of the classical subtypes of the disease. The follicular lymphoma and the Hodgkin lymphoma may occur together in the same biopsy, or in separate synchronous or metachronous biopsies.

IMMUNOHISTOCHEMISTRY

The tumour cells express surface, and often cytoplasmic, immunoglobulin showing light-chain restriction. IgM is the commonest heavy-chain isotype expressed. Surface immunoglobulin can be detected in frozen-section immunohistochemistry but is difficult to detect in paraffin sections because of the large amount of extracellular immunoglobulin present in most follicles. The detection of cytoplasmic immunoglobulin in paraffin sections requires good fixation and good technique.

The B-cell-associated antigens CD20 and CD79a are expressed. The tumour cells are negative for CD5, CD23 and CD43. Many follicular lymphomas express CD10, which serves to differentiate them from other low-grade B-cell lymphomas. Positive staining for CD45RA (MT2) may help to distinguish neoplastic from reactive follicles.

Approximately 85 per cent of follicular lymphomas express bcl-2 protein, more commonly in grade 1 than in grade 3 tumours. This is a particularly valuable marker because, in reactive follicle centre cells, bcl-2 is not expressed. Thus, bcl-2 provides a marker for the separation of reactive from neoplastic follicles. In interpreting bcl-2 staining, it should be noted that reactive T-cells, which are often abundant in neoplastic follicles, are bcl-2+. Ideally, a CD3 stain should be performed to determine the number and distribution of the T-cells, which should be distinguished from centrocytes in bcl-2-stained sections by their morphology. It should also be recognized that bcl-2 staining may be subtle, requiring a careful search for cytoplasmic positivity in perhaps only a proportion of the tumour cells. This contrasts with the total negativity of reactive follicle centre cells. Not all follicular lymphomas that express bcl-2 have the 14;18 translocation. Both neoplastic and reactive follicle centre cells express nuclear bcl-6.

GENETICS

Follicular lymphoma is characterized by the t(14;18) (q32;q21) translocation involving the immunoglobulin heavy-chain gene on chromosome 14 and the BCL-2 gene on chromosome 18. This translocation occurs in greater than 80 per cent of follicle centre cell lymphomas, in 20 per cent of diffuse large B-cell lymphomas and in 1–2 per cent of B-CLL. t(14;18) has also been found in B-cells of normal individuals. Other genetic events, including mutations of p53, are associated with tumour progression.

Table 5.2: Morphological differentiation between reactive and neoplastic follicular proliferations

REACTIVE	NEOPLASTIC
Follicles mainly distributed in cortex of node. Sinus structure of node usually identifiable	Closely packed follicles distributed throughout node. Sinus structure of node not usually identifiable
Follicles in perinodal tissues unusual	Follicles extending into perinodal and intranodal fat may be present
Mantle zone of small lymphocytes around follicles usually prominent	Mantle zone usually attenuated and may not be identifiable
Follicles of variable size; may show considerable variation in shape	Follicles of relatively uniform size and shape
Distribution of centroblasts and centrocytes zonal	Distribution of centroblasts and centrocytes random
Centroblasts form a large component of the follicle	Centroblasts usually form a minority population in the follicle and, in Grade 1, follicular lymphoma are scanty
Tingible body macrophages containing apoptotic debris often prominent	Tingible body macrophages usually absent
Centroblasts and centrocytes usually have typical morphology	Serpiginous, multinucleated and multilobated centroblasts may be present in the follicles and in the interfollicular zones.

Follicular lymphomas show clonal rearrangements of the immunoglobulin genes with a high level of ongoing mutations suggestive of antigen drive. Approximately 5 per cent of follicular lymphomas do not express immunoglobulin, in some cases owing to mutations that have introduced stop codons into the immunoglobulin genes. Such cases are presumably not responsive to antigen drive.

DIFFERENTIAL DIAGNOSIS

The main differential diagnosis of follicular lymphoma is with reactive follicular hyperplasia. The morphological features that aid the distinction between these two conditions are shown in Table 5.2. This differentiation is aided by immunohistochemical staining for bcl-2, CD45RA (MT2) and the proliferation marker Ki67. Apart from intrafollicular T-cells, reactive follicles are negative for bcl-2. Reactive follicles show a much higher proliferation fraction than most neoplastic follicles. Ki67 staining also highlights the zonal distribution of centroblasts in reactive follicles.

Small lymphocytic lymphoma with prominent proliferation centres may mimic follicular lymphoma. Morphologically the delicate nuclear structure of prolymphocytes and paraimmunoblasts can usually be differentiated from centroblasts and centrocytes. Immunohistochemistry shows the cells of small lymphocytic lymphoma to be CD5 and CD23+; follicle centre cells are negative for these two markers, although CD23

▲ **BOX 5.10: Follicular lymphoma: clinical features**

- ▲ 35 per cent of all non-Hodgkin lymphomas in USA; smaller percentage in the rest of the world
- ▲ Median age 59 years
- ▲ Male to female ratio 1:1.7
- ▲ Usually presents with stage III or IV disease
- ▲ Sites of involvement:
    Lymph nodes
    Bone marrow
    Peripheral blood
    Spleen
    Waldeyer's ring
- ▲ Primary follicular lymphomas of the gastro-intestinal tract and skin are clinically different from nodal follicular lymphomas

● BOX 5.11: Follicular lymphoma: morphology

- Loss of lymph node architecture
- Follicles composed of a mixture of centroblasts and centrocytes
- Regular-shaped follicles throughout node
- Attenuated mantle zones
- Follicles poorly defined
- Sclerosis common
- Grade 1, >5 blasts per high power field (HPF); grade 2, 6–15 blasts per HPF; grade 3, >15 blasts per HPF
- Grade 3A centroblasts and centrocytes present, grade 3B centroblasts only
  Growth patterns:
  Follicular > 75 per cent follicular
  Follicular and diffuse 25–75 per cent follicular
  Minimally follicular < 25 per cent follicular
- Variants (see text)

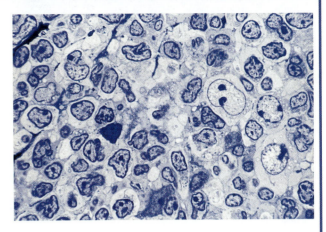

FIGURE 5.28 Plastic-embedded section of follicular lymphoma showing centrocytes and three centroblasts.

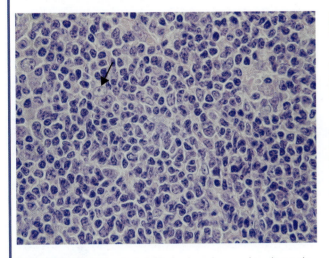

FIGURE 5.26 Grade 1 follicular lymphoma showing a single centroblast. The nucleus adjacent to the centroblast (arrow) is of a dendritic reticulum cell.

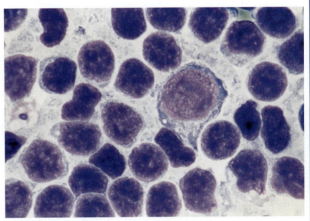

FIGURE 5.29 Imprint cytology of a grade 1 follicular lymphoma showing centrocytes and a centroblast.

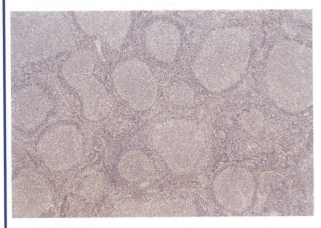

FIGURE 5.27 Follicular lymphoma. Relatively uniform follicles with attenuated mantles. No sinus structures seen.

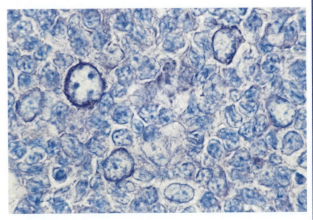

FIGURE 5.30 Follicular lymphoma. Giemsa stain showing basophilia of centroblast cytoplasm.

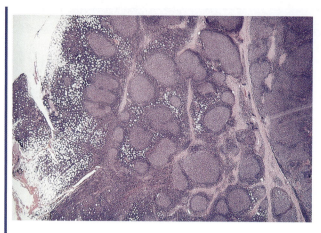

FIGURE 5.31 Follicular lymphoma showing extension into perinodal fat.

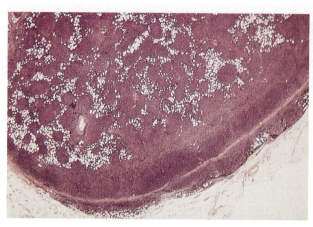

FIGURE 5.32 Follicular lymphoma involving axillary lymph node. Neoplastic follicles have invaded the fatty hilum and also extend outside the capsule.

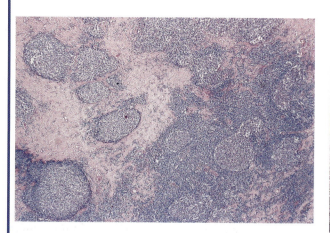

FIGURE 5.33 Follicular lymphoma showing sclerosis around follicles.

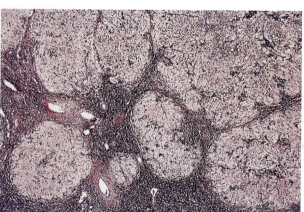

FIGURE 5.34 Follicular lymphoma showing sclerosis of follicle centres.

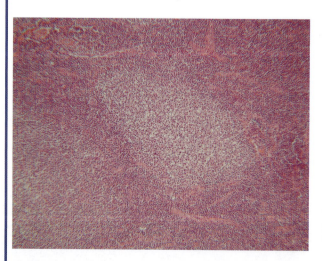

FIGURE 5.35 Follicular lymphoma showing signet ring change. Many of the cells appear vacuolated in this variant of follicular lymphoma.

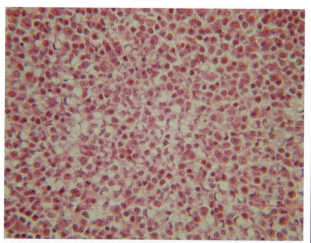

FIGURE 5.36 Follicular lymphoma showing signet ring change. The nucleus of many of the tumour cells is compressed to form a small crescent.

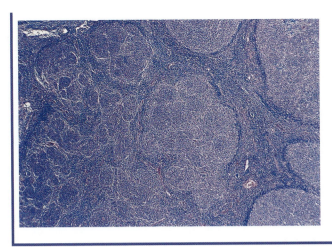

FIGURE 5.37 Follicular lymphoma in which one neoplastic follicle displays a floret pattern.

◆ **BOX 5.12: Follicular lymphoma: immunohistochemistry**

- ◆ Surface/cytoplasmic IgM+
- ◆ Surface/cytoplasmic IgD > IgG > IgA may be positive
- ◆ CD45RA (MT2)+
- ◆ CD10, CD20, CD79a+
- ◆ Bcl-6+
- ◆ Bcl-2+; grade 1, 100 per cent; grade 3, 75 per cent
- ◆ CD21 and CD23 identify dendritic cell networks

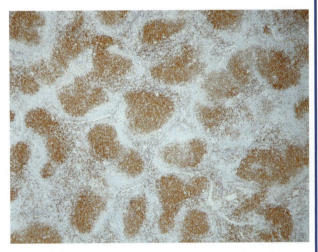

FIGURE 5.39 Grade 1 follicular lymphoma showing CD10 staining of follicle centre cells.

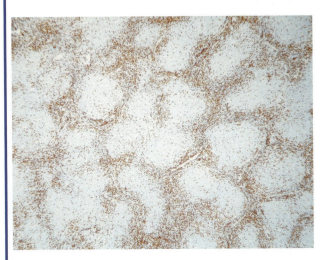

FIGURE 5.38 Follicular lymphoma showing follicles outlined by CD3-positive T-cells.

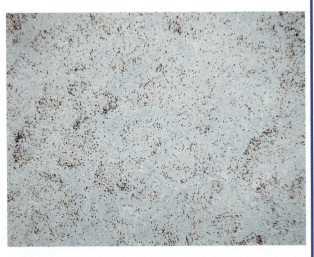

FIGURE 5.40 Grade 1 follicular lymphoma labelled for Ki67 showing a relatively low proliferation fraction. Note that many of the follicles show most labelling at the periphery.

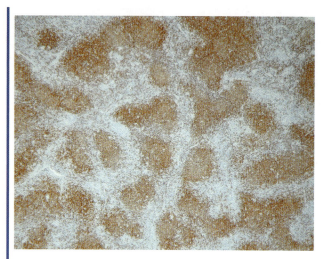

FIGURE 5.41 Follicular lymphoma stained for CD79a. The small dark cells are mantle cells that form attenuated mantles.

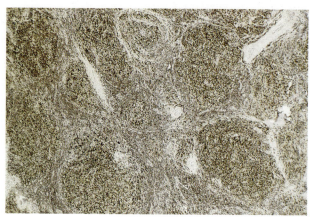

FIGURE 5.42 Follicular lymphoma stained for BCL-2 showing positivity of the follicle centres.

will label the dendritic cell network in the neoplastic follicles. Follicle centre cells are labelled by CD10 and show nuclear positivity for bcl-6; small lymphocytic lymphomas are negative for these markers.

Mantle cell lymphomas surround and colonize reactive germinal centres and often have a nodular structure. Residual reactive centroblasts at the centre of these nodules may heighten the resemblance to follicular lymphoma. The tumour cells of mantle cell lymphoma show CD5 positivity and express nuclear cyclin D1, which is almost pathognomic.

Nodal marginal zone lymphomas can be differentiated from follicular lymphomas on the basis that the follicles are reactive and have the morphological and immunohistochemical characteristics of reactive follicles. If they become totally colonized by tumour cells, in contrast to follicle centre cells, these will be CD10 and bcl-6 negative.

MANTLE CELL LYMPHOMA

Mantle cell lymphoma, previously obfuscated by the use of several synonyms (intermediate, mantle zone, centrocytic lymphoma, etc.), is now recognized as a well-defined entity (Banks *et al.* 1992). It frequently involves extranodal tissues, particularly the oropharynx and gastrointestinal tract, where it may present as lymphomatous polyposis. Peripheral lymphadenopathy is, however, the commonest presentation. High-stage disease with infiltration of the spleen and involvement of the bone marrow is common. Tumour cells may be found in the peripheral blood of such cases. Orchard *et al.* (2003) studied 80 cases of mantle cell lymphoma of which 37 had blood and bone marrow involvement with no evidence of nodal disease. Six of the latter group were long-term survivors. Five of this group had mutated immunoglobulin genes.

Mantle cell lymphomas frequently show a nodular growth pattern. This is due to their propensity to surround and replace pre-existing reactive germinal centres. Partially replaced germinal centres may be seen at the centre of tumour nodules. Their presence may be highlighted by immunohistochemistry, being bcl-2 negative in contrast with the positivity of the tumour cells, and showing a high proliferation index in contrast with the usual low proliferation index of the tumour cells.

The tumour cells of mantle cell lymphoma typically have oval or angulated nuclei, which frequently exhibit small clefts. The nuclear chromatin is granular and nucleoli are small and insignificant. In some cases, owing to intrinsic features of the tumour cells or to poor fixation, the tumour cells have rounded nuclei and distinction from small lymphocytic lymphoma may be difficult. The cytoplasm of the tumour cells is usually scanty and poorly defined. It is pale pink in H&E-stained sections and is weakly basophilic in Giemsa preparations.

The blood vessels in mantle cell lymphoma are often surrounded by hyaline basement membrane material. Reticulin stains highlight this material and may show spiky reticulin projections amongst the tumour cells. Another characteristic finding is the presence of histiocytes with large oval nuclei and abundant strongly eosinophilic cytoplasm.

There is a blastoid variant of mantle cell lymphoma in which the tumour cells have more open and finely granular nuclear chromatin. These tumours closely mimic lymphoblastic lymphomas. Rare pleomorphic (sarcomatoid) tumours occur. Proliferation indices, as measured by mitotic figures or immunohistochemistry, are variable in mantle cell lymphoma but tend to be higher in the blastoid and sarcomatoid forms.

IMMUNOHISTOCHEMISTRY

The tumour cells express surface immunoglobulin, usually IgM together with IgD. Cytoplasmic immunoglobulin and plasma cell differentiation are not seen. The B-cell antigens CD20 and CD79a are expressed, as are CD5 and CD43. In contrast to B-CLL, CD23 is not usually expressed on the tumour cells but labels the expanded network of dendritic cells. Immunohistochemical detection of cyclin D1 in the nuclei of tumour cells provides an almost specific marker for the identification of mantle cell lymphoma. It must be stressed that the expression of cyclin D1 must be in the nucleus, not the cytoplasm or nucleus and cytoplasm, which indicate artefactual staining. Endothelial cells provide a positive internal control for cyclin D1 staining.

GENETICS

Mantle cell lymphomas are characterized by the translocation t(11;14)(q13;q32), which brings the cyclin D1 gene on chromosome 11 under promoter influence of the immunoglobulin heavy-chain gene on chromosome 14. Cyclin D1, together with cyclin-dependent kinase (CDK4), phosphorylates retinoblastoma protein (pRB) releasing transcription factors that allow transition from the G1 to the S phase of the cell cycle. In the normal cell, p16/CDKN2 suppresses the cyclin D1/CDK4 phosphorylation of pRB. Deletions of the gene for p16/CDKN2 are associated with progression of mantle cell lymphoma and are positively correlated with proliferative activity of the tumour. Mantle cell lymphomas may show mutated or unmutated immunoglobulin genes.

▲ **BOX 5.13: Mantle cell lymphoma: clinical features**

- ▲ 3–10 per cent of all non-Hodgkin lymphomas
- ▲ Median age 60 years
- ▲ Male predominance, 2:1
- ▲ Usually present with stage III or IV disease
- ▲ Sites of involvement:
   Lymph nodes
   Bone marrow
   Peripheral blood
   Spleen
   Waldeyer's ring
   Gastrointestinal tract (lymphomatous polyposis)

● **BOX 5.14: Mantle cell lymphoma: morphology**

- Loss of normal lymph node architecture
- Tumour cells surround and infiltrate reactive germinal centres giving:
   Mantle zone growth pattern
   Nodular growth pattern
   Diffuse growth pattern
- Small to medium-sized cells with angulated nuclei. May be more rounded in some cases
- Nucleoli inconspicuous
- No paraimmunoblasts or neoplastic centroblasts
- Do not show plasma cell differentiation
- Blood vessels surrounded by hyaline basement membrane
- Characteristic histiocytes in some cases
- Blastoid variant (uncommon)

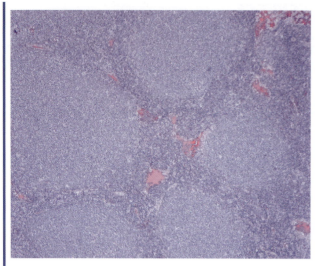

FIGURE 5.43 Mantle cell lymphoma showing a nodular growth pattern.

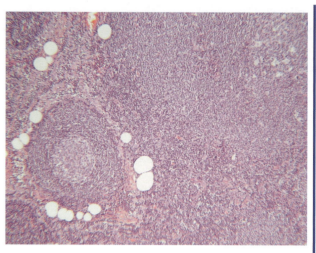

FIGURE 5.44 Mantle cell lymphoma showing a reactive follicle surrounded by tumour cells (lower left), a second follicle engulfed and infiltrated by tumour is seen upper right.

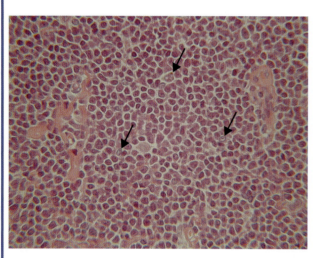

FIGURE 5.45 Mantle cell lymphoma showing characteristic perivascular hyaline material. Arrows indicate the nuclei of dispersed follicular dendritic cells.

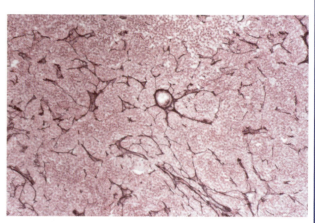

FIGURE 5.46 Mantle cell lymphoma stained for reticulin. Note condensation of reticulin around blood vessel with short radiating spikes.

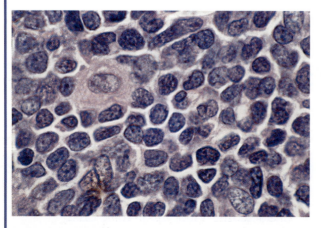

FIGURE 5.47 Mantle cell lymphoma showing characteristic cytomorphology. Note the characteristic histiocyte.

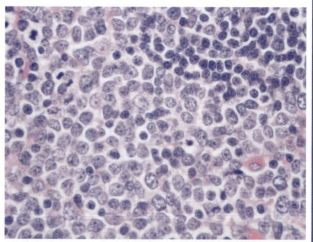

FIGURE 5.48 Blastic variant of mantle cell lymphoma. The tumour cells contrast in size with those of the usual type, seen upper right. The nuclear size, fine chromatin and visible (but small) nucleoli mimic the appearance of lymphoblastic lymphoma.

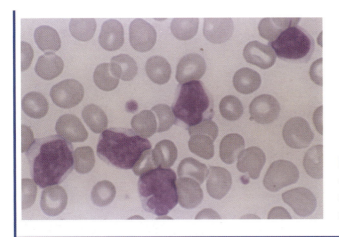

FIGURE 5.49 Blood film from a patient with mantle cell lymphoma. The circulating tumour cells show characteristic cleft nuclei with visible nucleoli and pale staining cytoplasm.

◆ **BOX 5.15: Mantle cell lymphoma: immunohistochemistry**

- Surface IgM+
- Surface IgD (usually) +
- CD5, CD20, CD79a+
- Nuclear cyclin D1 (bcl-1)+
- CD10−
- Bcl-6−
- CD21 and CD23 show expanded dendritic cell network

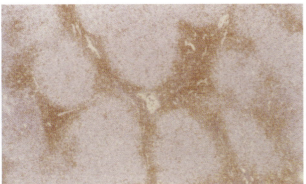

FIGURE 5.50 Nodular growth pattern of a mantle cell lymphoma highlighted by CD3+ T-cells.

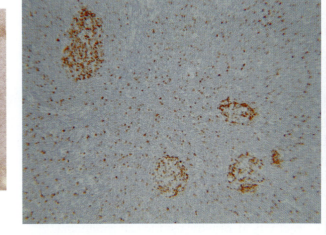

FIGURE 5.52 Mantle cell lymphoma stained for Ki67, showing a low proliferation fraction. The areas of intense labelling are residual reactive germinal centres.

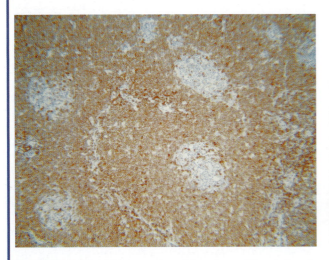

FIGURE 5.51 CD5+ mantle cell lymphoma. The dark cells are reactive T-lymphocytes. The unstained islands are residual reactive germinal centres surrounded by lymphoma.

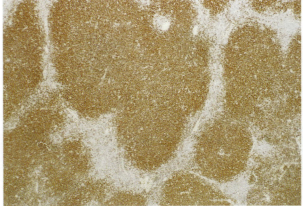

FIGURE 5.53 Mantle cell lymphoma stained for CD20 showing a nodular growth pattern.

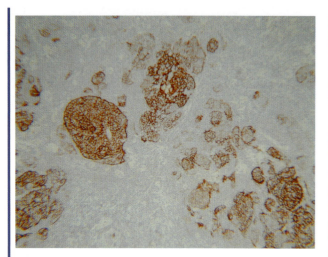

FIGURE 5.54 Mantle cell lymphoma stained for CD23 showing the characteristic expansion and dispersal of follicular dendritic cells.

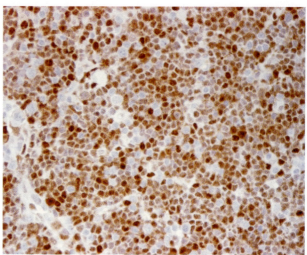

FIGURE 5.55 Mantle cell lymphoma stained for cyclin D1. Note that the staining is nuclear and varies in intensity.

DIFFERENTIAL DIAGNOSIS

The differentiation between mantle cell lymphoma and B-lymphocytic lymphoma can be difficult. This is an important differentiation since mantle cell lymphomas have a poor prognosis in comparison with all other small B-cell lymphomas. Morphologically, the identification of paraimmunoblasts, either singly or in proliferation centres identifies lymphocytic lymphoma. Proliferation centres must be differentiated from the remains of reactive germinal centres that may be found in mantle cell lymphomas. Conclusive separation may be obtained by immunohistochemistry, with CD23 positivity identifying lymphocytic lymphoma and cyclin D1 reactivity identifying mantle cell lymphoma.

Mantle cell lymphomas that have a nodular growth pattern may be mistaken for follicular lymphomas, especially if they have residual reactive centroblasts within the nodules. Mantle cell lymphoma cells (CD5+, cyclin D1+) can be distinguished from follicle centre cells (CD10+, bcl-6+) using immunohistochemistry.

The distinction between the blastic variant of mantle cell lymphoma and lymphoblastic lymphoma on morphological criteria can be difficult. Immunophenotypically, the distinction is clear-cut with lymphoblastic lymphomas displaying an immature T- or B-cell phenotype and expressing terminal deoxynucleotidyl transferase (TdT) but not cyclin D1.

DIFFUSE LARGE B-CELL LYMPHOMA

Diffuse large B-cell lymphoma (DLBCL) encompasses all B-cell lymphomas with a diffuse growth pattern and cells more than twice the size of small lymphocytes. It accounts for approximately 40 per cent of adult B-cell non-Hodgkin lymphomas and has a wide age range with a median in the seventh decade. Involvement of extranodal sites occurs in 40 per cent of cases, frequently as primary tumours. DLBCL usually appear to arise *de novo* but may follow transformation of a pre-existing low-grade B-cell lymphoma.

Diffuse large B-cell lymphoma is not a homogeneous group of tumours. Apart from the fact that some appear

to be primary and others evolve from pre-existing low-grade B-cell lymphomas, four morphological subtypes (centroblastic, immunoblastic, T-cell-rich large B-cell lymphoma and anaplastic) are recognized in the WHO classification. It has also been shown that DLBCL can be subdivided on the basis of their gene expression profiles into those resembling germinal centre B-cells and those resembling activated B-cells, with the former having a better prognosis than the latter (Alizadeh *et al.* 2000). Immunohistochemistry is being used increasingly to detect the products of genes that have been shown by DNA microarrays to have prognostic significance, and thus to divide DLBCL into good and bad prognostic subgroups (Rosenwald *et al.* 2002, Rimsza *et al.* 2004).

CENTROBLASTIC LYMPHOMA

Centroblasts have rounded nuclei, open nuclear chromatin and two to five nucleoli that often appear to be attached to the nuclear membrane. They have basophilic cytoplasm. Lennert and co-workers (Hui *et al.* 1988) recognized four morphological variants of centroblastic lymphoma cells: monomorphic, multilobated, centrocytoid and polymorphic. Although the centrocytoid variant described has subsequently been interpreted as the blastic variant of mantle cell lymphoma, it may be worth retaining the term 'centrocytoid' for the large and small serpiginous cells often seen in follicular lymphomas and DLBCL. This morphological variation is not known to have any biological or clinical significance, although primary large B-cell lymphomas of bone are reported to be composed predominantly of the multilobated subtype. Histopathologists should, however, be familiar with these subtypes, since their recognition can aid the histological diagnosis of centroblastic lymphoma and its separation from other neoplasms.

Monomorphic centroblastic lymphoma is composed of uniform cells as described above. Multilobated centroblasts exhibit lobated nuclei, fine nuclear chromatin and inconspicuous nucleoli. Centrocytoid centroblasts have elongated, sometimes serpiginous nuclei within which nucleoli are visible. The polymorphic subtype may contain all of these variants as well as immunoblasts and more pleomorphic, often multinucleated, cells.

IMMUNOBLASTIC LYMPHOMA

Immunoblasts have round or oval nuclei with a prominent central nucleolus. Their cytoplasm is deeply basophilic. Cells with this morphology are seen within a high proportion of centroblastic lymphomas and may account for up to 90 per cent of the tumour cells. It was for this reason that centroblastic and immunoblastic lymphomas were merged into the single category of diffuse large B-cell lymphoma in the WHO classification. However, immunoblastic lymphoma was also a term used to categorize tumours that resulted from the transformation of immunocytomas (lymphoplasmacytic lymphomas). Further studies are needed to determine whether immunoblastic lymphoma (a tumour composed of more than 90 per cent immunoblasts) is a clinicopathological entity or should remain as a morphological variant of diffuse large B-cell lymphoma.

T-CELL/HISTIOCYTE-RICH LARGE B-CELL LYMPHOMA

T-cell/histiocyte-rich large B-cell lymphoma (T/HRLBCL) is categorized as a morphological variant of DLBCL in the WHO classification. The tumour has a background of sheets of small T-cells with a variable mixture of histiocytes (often epithelioid) diffusely spread or forming loose aggregates. The tumour cells (large B-cells) are scattered uniformly, with occasional small clusters, throughout the infiltrate. The tumour cells should constitute less than 10 per cent of the total cellular population. Small B-lymphocytes are absent or scarce. The overall growth pattern of the tumour is diffuse.

A recently reported study of 30 cases of T/HRLBCL found three morphological subtypes in which the large B-cells resembled either the 'popcorn' cells of lymphocyte-predominant Hodgkin lymphoma, centroblasts and immunoblasts or classic Reed–Sternberg cells (Lim *et al.* 2002). There were clinical and immunohistochemical differences between these groups, suggesting that T/HRLBCL may be a heterogeneous category. The tumour cells show mutated immunoglobulin genes and usually express bcl-6, suggesting germinal centre origin. However, in contrast to most follicular lymphomas, they do not usually express CD10 or bcl-2, and t(14;18) is rarely identified.

The main differential diagnosis for T/HRLBCL is with lymphocyte-predominant Hodgkin lymphoma (Table 5.3). In a study of 139 cases of nodular lymphocyte-predominant Hodgkin lymphoma (NLPHL) and 79 cases of T/HRLBCL, Boudova *et al.* (2003) found that, while the tumour cells of both entities were immunophenotypically similar, in NLPHL small B-cells and CD3+, CD4+, CD57+ T-cells were common, in T/HRLBCL, CD8+ T-cells and histiocytes predominated. Expanded networks of follicular dendritic cells were found in NLPHL but were absent in T/HRLBCL. Comparative genomic hybridization has shown differences between T/HRLBCL and NLPHL (Franke *et al.* 2002).

ANAPLASTIC LYMPHOMA

This is an uncommon variant of DLBCL (not to be confused with the pleomorphic variant of centroblastic lymphoma). The tumour cells are large with abundant cytoplasm and atypical nuclei. They are often multinucleated and may resemble Reed–Sternberg cells, but not the hallmark cells of cytotoxic T-cell-derived anaplastic large cell lymphoma. The tumour cells are positive for one or more B-cell markers and CD30, but do not express ALK protein (Haralambieva *et al.* 2000). The cells often grow in a cohesive fashion and show sinusoidal permeation.

DIFFUSE LARGE B-CELL LYMPHOMA WITH EXPRESSION OF ALK

This is a rare variant of DLBCL. The tumour cells resemble immunoblasts or plasmablasts, but have more abundant basophilic (amphophilic) cytoplasm. The tumour cells do not express B-cell antigens and are CD30−. They express cytoplasmic IgA and show granular cytoplasmic positivity for the ALK protein. Some tumours show the t(2;17)(p23;q23) translocation involving the ALK gene at chromosome band 2p23 and the clathrin gene at chromosome band 17q23 (De Paepe *et al.* 2003, Gascoyne *et al.* 2003). The tumour shows a male predominance may occur in childhood and follows an aggressive course. Two paediatric patients have been described with ALK-positive plasmablastic B-cell lymphomas expressing the t(2;5) *NPM-ALK* fusion transcript characteristic of many T-null-cell anaplastic large cell lymphomas (Onciu *et al.* 2003).

IMMUNOHISTOCHEMISTRY

The cells of DLBCL express CD45 and B-cell markers, of which CD20 and CD79a are most commonly used.

Most tumours express surface and/or cytoplasmic immunoglobulin, although this will be difficult to detect in poorly fixed specimens in which diffusion artefacts can make interpretation difficult. Immunoglobulin inclusions may be seen. Cells of the anaplastic variant are CD30+. In other DLBCLs, occasional cells, particularly giant cell forms, may express CD30. Approximately 10 per cent of DLBCL express CD5, but this does not imply a relationship to CLL/SLL or mantle cell lymphoma; cyclin D1 is negative in these cases. A larger proportion expresses CD10, which probably indicates follicle centre cell derivation. Approximately half the cases express bcl-2; this has no diagnostic significance but may be an adverse prognostic factor. In a large proportion of DLCBL, more than 10 per cent of the tumour cells express nuclear bcl-6. The proliferation fraction, as determined by Ki67 staining, ranges from 30 to over 90 per cent.

GENETICS

Most DLCBL have a postgerminal centre genotype with rearrangement of the immunoglobulin genes and mutated v-region genes. Approximately one-third of cases show t(14;18), probably indicating evolution from follicle centre cell lymphoma. Another third shows translocations and other abnormalities of 3q27 involving the BCL-6 gene. Many cases show a complex genotype with multiple abnormalities. Reference has already been made to the observation that DLBCL with a gene expression profile resembling germinal centre cells have a better prognosis than those having a profile resembling activated B-cells.

Table 5.3: Differential diagnosis between T-cell/histiocyte-rich large B-cell lymphoma (T/HRLBCL) and nodular lymphocyte-predominant Hodgkin lymphoma (NLPHL)

	T/HRLBCL	NLPHL
Growth pattern	Diffuse	Nodular or nodular and diffuse
Tumour cell morphology	Centroblasts, less commonly L & H cells or Reed–Sternberg cells	L & H cells
T-cell rosetting of tumour cells	No	Yes
CD30	Some positive	Negative
Background reactive cells	Mostly CD8-positive T-cell and histiocytes	Variable small B-cells. CD3, CD4, CD57-positive T-cells
Nodular meshwork of dendritic cells	Absent	Present

'L & H cells' is the term commonly applied to the large neoplastic B-cells (popcorn cells) in NLPHL.

DIFFERENTIAL DIAGNOSIS

Diffuse large B-cell lymphoma can usually be identified in good-quality histological preparations by the recognition of centroblasts, their variants and immunoblasts. A partially nodular growth pattern may indicate origin from a follicular lymphoma. DLBCL and its variants can be distinguished from melanoma and anaplastic carcinoma by immunohistochemistry. T-Cell histiocyte-rich large B-cell lymphoma presents the greatest problem in its differentiation from nodular lymphocyte-predominant Hodgkin lymphoma and, currently, there is a grey zone between these lymphomas (see Table 5.3).

MEDIASTINAL (THYMIC) LARGE B-CELL LYMPHOMA

Mediastinal large B-cell lymphoma (MLBCL), a tumour thought to be derived from thymic B-cells, is recognized as a subtype of DLBCL in the WHO classification. It usually presents with symptoms and signs of an anterior mediastinal mass. Dissemination occurs to the kidney, adrenal, liver, skin and brain, but lymph node involvement is rarely encountered. Morphologically, the tumour differs from other DLBCL in that the tumour cells often have clear cytoplasm and they may be compartmentalized by fine sclerosis.

IMMUNOHISTOCHEMISTRY

The tumour cells express CD45 and B-cell markers. They do not express CD5 or CD10. Immunoglobulin and HLA molecules are often undetectable. CD30 is often expressed.

GENETICS

Immunoglobulin genes are rearranged. Genetic abnormalities that characterize other types of DLBCL are absent. Abnormal expression of the *REL* gene and the *MAL* gene has been reported in a large number of cases. Recent studies have shown that the gene expression profile of MLBCL differs from that of other DLBCL and

has features in common with classic Hodgkin lymphoma (Savage *et al.* 2003). Immunohistochemical detection of nuclear phosphorylated STAT6, a feature shared by MLBCL and cHL, may aid the differentiation between MLBCL and other subtypes of DLBCL (Guiter *et al.* 2004).

DIFFERENTIAL DIAGNOSIS

The differential diagnosis between MLBCL and other types of DLBCL in a mediastinal biopsy may be difficult. The presence of thymic remnants, clear cells and/or sclerosis will favour MLBCL. In the absence of these features, immunophenotypic and genetic characteristics may aid the differentiation, in particular, detection of MAL protein or STAT6.

INTRAVASCULAR LARGE B-CELL LYMPHOMA

Intravascular large B-cell lymphoma is recognized as a rare subtype of DLBCL in the WHO classification. The tumour cells appear to lack certain adhesion molecules and in biopsies are seen within the lumina of small blood vessels. The presentation of the tumour is at extranodal sites and lymph node involvement is unlikely to be encountered.

> ▲ **BOX 5.16: Diffuse large B-cell lymphoma: clinical features**
>
> ▲ 30–40 per cent of adult non-Hodgkin lymphomas
> ▲ May occur at all ages; median age seventh decade
> ▲ Slight male predominance
> ▲ 60 per cent nodal, 40 per cent extranodal
> ▲ May be primary or may represent transformation of a low-grade B-cell lymphoma

> ● **BOX 5.17: Diffuse large B-cell lymphoma: morphology**
>
> - Tumour cells at least twice the size of small lymphocytes
> - Various morphological forms: immunoblasts, centroblasts (monomorphic, multilobated, centrocytoid, polymorphic) in varying proportions
> - Partial or complete effacement of nodal architecture
> - Sinusoidal pattern of infiltration uncommon
> - Variable admixed T-cell and/or histiocytes
> - Variable sclerosis

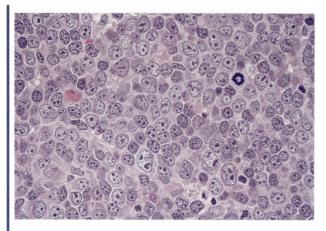

FIGURE 5.56 Diffuse large B-cell lymphoma (centroblastic monomorphic).

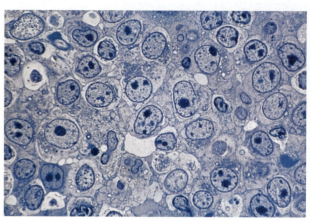

FIGURE 5.57 Diffuse large B-cell lymphoma (centroblastic monomorphic). Plastic-embedded section.

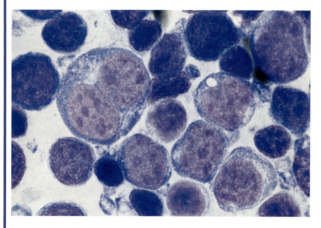

FIGURE 5.58 Diffuse large B-cell lymphoma (centroblastic). Imprint preparation showing moderate pleomorphism.

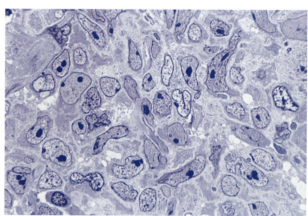

FIGURE 5.59 Diffuse large B-cell lymphoma (centroblastic centrocytoid). Plastic-embedded section showing large centrocytoid cells with prominent nucleoli.

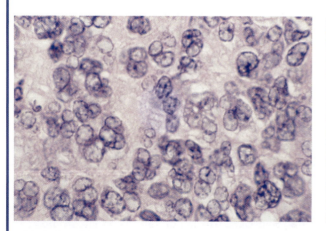

FIGURE 5.60 Diffuse large B-cell lymphoma (centroblastic multilobated).

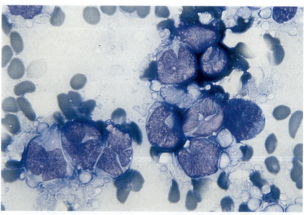

FIGURE 5.61 Diffuse large B-cell lymphoma (centroblastic multilobated). Imprint preparation.

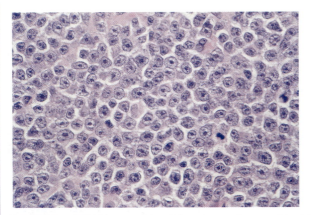

FIGURE 5.62 Diffuse large B-cell lymphoma (immunoblastic).

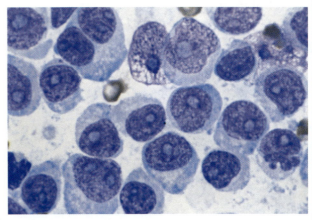

FIGURE 5.63 Diffuse large B-cell lymphoma (immunoblastic). Imprint preparation.

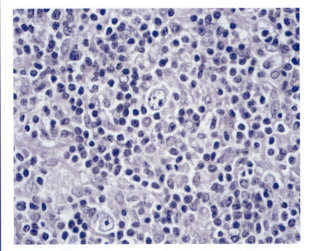

FIGURE 5.64 T-cell/histiocyte-rich B-cell lymphoma showing a tumour cell with centroblast morphology. The surrounding cells are predominantly T-cells and histiocytes.

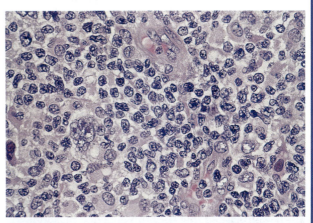

FIGURE 5.65 T-cell/histiocyte-rich diffuse large B-cell lymphoma with a tumour cell resembling a Reed–Sternberg cell.

◆ BOX 5.18: Diffuse large B-cell lymphoma: immunohistochemistry

- ◆ CD20 and CD79a+
- ◆ Surface and/or cytoplasmic immunoglobulin IgM > IgG > IgA
- ◆ Approximately 10 per cent of cases are CD5+
- ◆ 25–50 per cent of cases are CD10+

- ◆ 30–50 per cent of cases are bcl-2+
- ◆ Many cases are bcl-6+
- ◆ CD30+ in anaplastic variant, occasional cells positive in many cases
- ◆ Ki67 labelling fraction 40–90 per cent

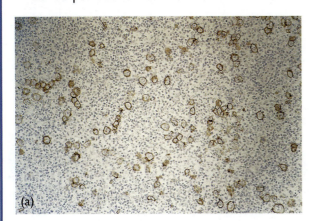

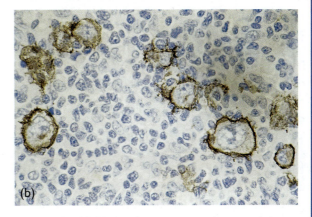

FIGURE 5.66 T-cell/histiocyte-rich diffuse large B-cell lymphoma stained for CD20 showing strong membrane staining of the tumour cells. (a) Low power; (b) high power.

BURKITT LYMPHOMA/LEUKAEMIA

Denis Burkitt, while working as a surgeon in Uganda, described a childhood tumour syndrome with characteristic clinico-anatomical features. This tumour appeared to be limited to the warm wet tropics of Africa and Papua New Guinea. A meeting of haematopathologists held in 1968 under the auspices of the WHO proposed that this tumour should be defined by its cytology and histology. Using this definition, it became apparent that Burkitt lymphoma (BL) was not confined to the wet tropics but occurred sporadically throughout the world. In later years, a proportion of high-grade B-cell lymphomas occurring in patients with acquired immunodeficiency syndrome (AIDS) were found to have the cytological and histological features of Burkitt lymphoma.

Burkitt lymphoma may, therefore, be divided into three subtypes (endemic BL, sporadic BL and immunodeficiency-associated BL) with identical cytological and histological features, but different clinical and gross anatomical characteristics. The common cytomorphology of these tumours is related to the presence in all three subtypes of translocations between the c-myc oncogene and immunoglobulin genes that results in unrestrained cell proliferation without differentiation. It must be emphasized that the term endemic BL should be used for tumours with the characteristics described by Denis Burkitt and not for all tumours with the microscopic features of BL occurring in the wet tropics. AIDS is prevalent in the wet tropics and a proportion of cases occurring in these regions will be immunodeficiency associated, while rare cases may be of the sporadic type.

ENDEMIC BURKITT LYMPHOMA

Endemic BL is rare before the age of 2 years and has a peak incidence at age 7 years; the incidence after the age of 15 years is low. It has a male to female sex incidence of approximately 2:1. The most characteristic and best known feature of this tumour is the occurrence of one or, more commonly, multiple, jaw tumours. This feature is age dependent, and is almost certainly related to dental development and to the presence of cellular marrow in the jaws. All BL patients aged 3 years in Uganda were found to have jaw tumours, the proportion falling thereafter to 10 per cent at the age of 15 years. This accounts for the observation that the overall incidence of jaw tumours is in the region of 50 per cent, a proportion that will vary with the age of the patient population studied. Other common sites of involvement are brain (18 per cent), heart (32 per cent), stomach

(26 per cent), small intestine (28 per cent), liver (37 per cent), pancreas (43 per cent), kidney (77 per cent), ovaries (82 per cent of females), testis (12 per cent of males), thyroid (37 per cent) and adrenals (58 per cent). Intra-abdominal lymph nodes, often within retroperitoneal masses, are frequently involved; peripheral lymphadenopathy is uncommon. Massive bilateral breast involvement may occur in girls who are pregnant or lactating.

SPORADIC BURKITT LYMPHOMA

Burkitt lymphoma is the commonest non-Hodgkin lymphoma of children under the age of 15 years in the developed world. The tumour is also seen in young adults and, less commonly, in older age groups. It has a male predominance of 5:1 or more. It presents most commonly with intra-abdominal tumour, which often appears to have originated in the ileo-caecal region. Involvement of the lymphoid tissue of Waldeyer's ring is also seen. Both of these anatomical sites are rarely involved in endemic BL. Peripheral lymphadenopathy is seen more frequently than in endemic BL but is not common. Sporadic BL may also involve the kidneys, ovaries and breasts. Bone marrow involvement may be associated with leukaemic overspill into the peripheral blood. In a small proportion of sporadic cases in young children, the disease may closely resemble endemic BL in its distribution with jaw tumours and multiple visceral involvement. It is possible that these cases may have a similar aetiopathology to the endemic disease.

IMMUNODEFICIENCY-ASSOCIATED BURKITT LYMPHOMA

Burkitt lymphoma may present as nodal or extranodal disease in patients with AIDS and, in these patients, is often the initial manifestation of AIDS. It is an uncommon tumour in other forms of immunodeficiency.

MORPHOLOGY

Burkitt lymphoma is most easily diagnosed on imprint or other cytological preparations. Nuclei are rounded and may show clefts. The nuclear chromatin is finely granular and there are up to five visible, but not usually conspicuous, nucleoli. The cytoplasm is deeply basophilic with a paler area corresponding to the position of the

Golgi body. Cytoplasmic vacuolation caused by neutral fat droplets is characteristic but not always present.

Histologically, the tumour cells have rounded and relatively uniform nuclei that approximate the size of the nuclei of 'starry-sky' (tingible body) macrophages within the tumour. The nuclear chromatin appears granular. Two to five nucleoli are usually discernible, but are not usually prominent. The cytoplasm is best seen at the edge of the section where the cells tend to separate. It forms a well-defined rim around the nucleus, and appears amphophilic in H&E-stained sections and deeply basophilic in Giemsa-stained preparations. High-power microscopy will often reveal small vacuoles within this cytoplasmic rim. These fat droplets can be demonstrated in frozen sections of formalin-fixed tissue with neutral fat stains. They are characteristic but not specific for BL.

Burkitt lymphoma always shows a high mitotic index, and apoptotic nuclei and nuclear fragments are common. Many of these are engulfed within macrophages that give a characteristic 'starry-sky' pattern to the tumour.

The WHO classification includes a variant designated 'atypical Burkitt/Burkitt-like' lymphoma. This has morphological features of BL but shows greater degrees of pleomorphism. Such tumours probably have translocations resulting in c-myc deregulation. Even endemic BL may become pleomorphic in recurrences following chemotherapy to the extent of exhibiting Reed–Sternberg-like cells.

IMMUNOHISTOCHEMISTRY

The tumour cells express the B-cell antigens CD20 and CD79a. They also express CD10 and BCL-6, consistent with germinal centre cell origin but are BCL-2−. Staining for Ki-67 is diagnostically helpful since all BL cells are in cycle, as a consequence of c-myc deregulation; therefore, the labelling index of the viable tumour cells will be 100 per cent. Burkitt leukaemia, previously categorized as a type of lymphoblastic leukaemia, has a mature B-cell phenotype and is TdT−, in contrast to precursor B-cell leukaemia/lymphoma.

GENETICS

All types of BL show translocations between the c-myc oncogene on chromosome 8 and one of the immunoglobulin genes: usually the heavy-chain gene on chromosome 14, less commonly the κ-light-chain gene on chromosome 2 or the λ-light-chain gene on chromosome 22. There are subtle differences in the breakpoint region on chromosome 14 between endemic (joining region) and sporadic (switch region) BL.

Epstein–Barr virus genomes can be demonstrated in all cases of endemic BL. In sporadic BL, the incidence shows geographic variation, being approximately 30 per cent in the developed world, but 70–80 per cent in North Africa and South America. EBV genomes are

---

▲ **BOX 5.19: Burkitt lymphoma (BL)/ leukaemia: clinical features**

ENDEMIC BL
- Childhood predominance (median age 7 years)
- Male predominance 2:1
- Sites of involvement: jaws, gastrointestinal tract, kidneys, liver, pancreas, retroperitoneum, gonads, breast, endocrine organs, brain
- Leukaemic manifestations rare

SPORADIC BL
- Children and young adults
- Male predominance 5:1
- Sites of involvement: ileo-caecal region, abdomen and pelvis, Waldeyer's ring, peripheral lymph nodes
- Leukaemic manifestations uncommon

IMMUNODEFICIENCY-ASSOCIATED BL (ACQUIRED IMMUNE DEFICIENCY SYNDROME)
- Young adults
- Sites of involvement: nodal and extranodal

● **BOX 5.20: Burkitt lymphoma/leukaemia: morphology**

- Monomorphic small blast cells
- Defined basophilic (amphophilic) cytoplasm
- Cytoplasmic lipid droplets/vacuoles
- Proliferation index 100 per cent
- Numerous apoptotic bodies
- 'Starry-sky' macrophages

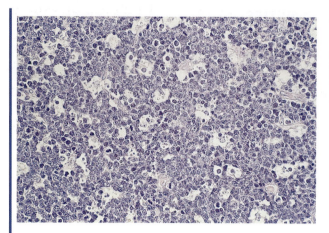

FIGURE 5.67 Burkitt lymphoma showing a 'starry-sky' pattern.

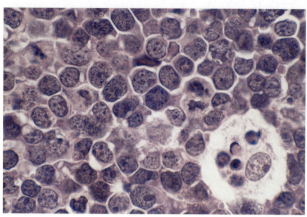

FIGURE 5.68 High-power view of Burkitt lymphoma showing characteristic morphology of the tumour cells.

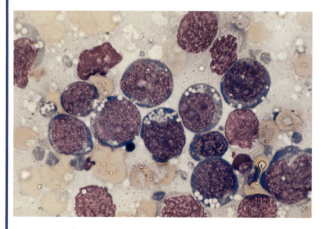

FIGURE 5.69 Endemic Burkitt lymphoma. Imprint showing characteristic tumour cells.

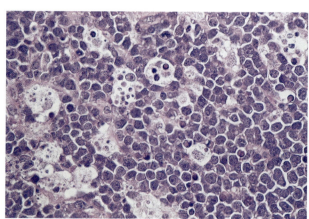

FIGURE 5.70 Burkitt lymphoma. Note apoptotic debris in 'starry-sky' macrophages.

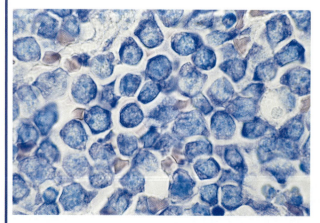

FIGURE 5.71 Burkitt lymphoma, stained with Giemsa, showing lipid vacuoles in deeply basophilic cytoplasm.

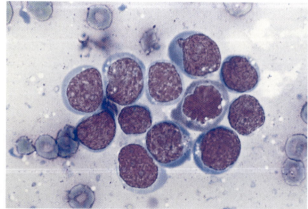

FIGURE 5.72 Sporadic Burkitt lymphoma. Imprint showing features similar to those of the endemic tumour.

◆ BOX 5.21: Burkitt lymphoma/leukaemia: immunohistochemistry

- ◆ Membrane immunoglobulin M (IgM) with light-chain restriction
- ◆ Do not express cytoplasmic Ig
- ◆ CD20 and CD79a+
- ◆ CD10+
- ◆ BCL-6+
- ◆ BCL-2−
- ◆ Terminal deoxynucleotidyl transferase (TdT) negative

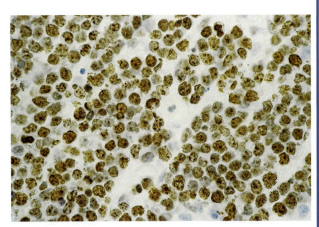

FIGURE 5.73 Burkitt lymphoma stained for Ki67, showing labelling of 100 per cent of the tumour cells.

exhibited by 25–40 per cent of immunodeficiency-associated BL.

DIFFERENTIAL DIAGNOSIS

The main differential diagnosis of BL is with diffuse large B-cell lymphomas that show a prominent 'starry-sky' pattern and a high proliferation fraction. Such tumours may be designated as atypical Burkitt/Burkitt-like lymphomas. The demonstration of uniform cytology, deep cytoplasmic basophilia and a proliferation index among viable cells of not less than 100 per cent favours a diagnosis of BL. There is a small grey area between BL and DLBCL, possibly as a consequence of translocations resulting in c-myc deregulation in a small proportion of DLBCL.

REFERENCES

Alizadeh AA, Eisen MB, Davis RE, *et al.* 2000 Distinct types of diffuse large B-cell lymphoma identified by gene expression profiling. *Nature* **403**: 503–511.

Andriko J-AW, Swerdlow SH, Aguilera NI, Abbondanzo SL 2001 Is lymphoplasmacytic lymphoma/immunocytoma a distinct entity? A clinicopathological study of 20 cases. *American Journal of Surgical Pathology* **25**: 742–751.

Asplund SL, McKenna RW, Howard M, Croft SH 2002 Immunophenotype does not correlate with lymph node histology in chronic lymphocytic leukemia/small lymphocytic lymphoma. *American Journal of Surgical Pathology* **26**: 624–629.

Ballesteros E, Osborne BM, Matushima AY 1998 CD5+ low grade marginal zone B-cell lymphomas with localized presentation. *American Journal of Surgical Pathology* **22**: 201–207.

Banks PM, Chan J, Cleary ML, *et al.* 1992 Mantle cell lymphoma. A proposal for unification of morphologic, immunologic and molecular data. *American Journal of Surgical Pathology* **16**: 637–640.

Bosga–Bouwer AG, van Imhoff GW, Boonstra R, *et al.* 2003 Follicular lymphoma grade 3B includes 3 cytogenetically defined subgroups with primary t(14;18), 3q27, or other translocations: t(14;18) and 3q27 are mutually exclusive. *Blood* **101**: 1149–1154.

Boudova L, Torlakovic E, Delabie J, *et al.* 2003 Nodular lymphocyte-predominant Hodgkin lymphoma with nodules resembling T-cell/histiocyte rich B-cell lymphoma: differential diagnosis between nodular lymphocyte-predominant Hodgkin lymphoma and T-cell/histiocyte rich B-cell lymphoma. *Blood* **102**: 3753–3758.

Camacho FI, Algara P, Mollejo M, *et al.* 2003 Nodal marginal zone lymphoma: a heterogeneous tumor. *American Journal of Surgical Pathology* **27**: 762–771.

Campo E, Miquel R, Krenacs L, *et al.* 1999. Primary nodal marginal zone lymphomas of splenic and MALT type. *American Journal of Surgical Pathology* **23**: 59–68.

Chang C-C, McClintock S, Cleveland RP, *et al.* 2004 Immunohistochemical expression patterns of germinal center and activation B-cell markers correlate with prognosis in diffuse large B-cell lymphoma. *American Journal of Surgical Pathology* **28**: 464–470.

De Paepe P, Baens M, van Krieken H, *et al.* 2003 ALK activation by the *CLTC-ALK* fusion is a recurrent event in large B-cell lymphoma. *Blood* **102**: 2638–2641.

Franke S, Wlodarska I, Maes B, *et al.* 2002 Comparative genomic hybridization pattern distinguishes T-cell/histiocyte rich B-cell lymphoma from nodular lymphocyte predominance Hodgkin's lymphoma. *American Journal of Pathology* **161**: 1861–1867.

Gascoyne RD, Lamant L, Martin-Subero JI, *et al.* 2003 ALK-positive diffuse large B-cell lymphoma is associated with *Clathrin–ALK* rearrangements: report of 6 cases. *Blood* **102**: 2568–2573.

Guiter C, Dusanter-Fourt I, Copie-Bergman C, *et al.* 2004 Constitutive STAT6 activation in primary mediastinal large B-cell lymphoma. *Blood* **104**: 543–549.

Haralambieva E, Pulford KAF, Lamant L, *et al.* 2000 Anaplastic large-cell lymphomas of B-cell phenotype are anaplastic lymphoma kinase (ALK) negative and belong to the spectrum of diffuse large B-cell lymphomas. *British Journal of Haematology* **109**: 584–591.

Hui PK, Feller AC, Lennert K 1988 High-grade non-Hodgkin's lymphoma of B-cell type. I. Histopathology. *Histopathology* **12**: 127–143.

Lim MS, Beaty M, Sorbara L, *et al.* 2002 T-cell/histiocyte-rich large B-cell lymphoma. A heterogeneous entity with derivation from germinal center B-cells. *American Journal of Surgical Pathology* **26**: 1458–1466.

Mann RB, Berard CW 1983 Criteria for the cytological subclassification of follicular lymphomas: a proposed alternative method. *Hematological Oncology* **1**: 187–192.

Onciu M, Behm FG, Downing JR, *et al.* 2003 ALK-positive plasmablastic B-cell lymphoma with expression of the NPM-ALK fusion transcript: report of 2 cases. *Blood* **102**: 2642–2644.

Orchard J, Garand R, Davis Z, *et al.* 2003 A subset of t(11;14) lymphoma with mantle cell features displays mutated IgVh genes and includes patients with good prognosis, nonnodal disease. *Blood* **101**: 4975–4981.

Rimsza LM, Roberts RA, Miller TP, *et al.* 2004 Loss of MHC class II gene and protein expression in diffuse large B-cell lymphoma is related to decreased tumor immunosurveillance and poor patient survival regardless of other prognostic factors: a follow-up study from the Leukemia and Lymphoma Molecular Profiling Project. *Blood* **103**: 4251–4258.

Rosenwald A, Wright G, Chan WC, *et al.* 2002 The use of molecular profiling to predict survival after chemotherapy for diffuse large B-cell lymphoma. *New England Journal of Medicine* **346**: 1937–1947.

Sanchez-Beato M, Sanchez-Aguilera A, Piris MA 2003 Cell cycle deregulation in B-cell lymphomas. *Blood* **101**: 1220–1235.

Savage KJ, Monti S, Kutok JL, *et al.* 2003 The molecular signature of mediastinal large B-cell lymphoma differs from that of other diffuse large B-cell lymphomas and shares features with classical Hodgkin lymphoma. *Blood* **102**: 3871–3879.

Sheibani K, Sohn CC, Burke JS, Winberg CD, Wu AM, Rappaport H 1986 Monocytoid B-cell lymphoma: a novel B-cell neoplasm. *American Journal of Pathology* **124**: 310–318.

Sheibani K, Burke JS, Swartz WG, *et al.* 1988 Monocytoid B-cell lymphoma: clinicopathologic study of 21 cases of a unique type of low-grade lymphoma. *Cancer* **62**: 1531–1538.

Thieblemont C, Nasser V, Felman P, *et al.* 2004 Small lymphocytic lymphoma, marginal zone B-cell lymphoma and mantle cell lymphoma exhibit distinct gene expression profiles allowing molecular diagnosis. *Blood* **103**: 2727–2737.

Weistner A, Rosenwald A, Barry TS, *et al.* 2003 ZAP-70 expression identifies a chronic lymphocytic leukemia subtype with unmutated immunoglobulin genes, inferior clinical outcome, and distinct gene expression profile. *Blood* **101**: 4944–4951.

6 T-CELL LYMPHOMAS

OVERVIEW

T-cell neoplasms are less common than B-cell lymphomas but their incidence shows both geographical and racial variations. In the International Non-Hodgkin Lymphoma Classification Study of cases from the USA, Europe, Asia and South Africa, peripheral T-cell lymphomas accounted for 7.6 per cent of the total with anaplastic large cell lymphoma forming an additional 2.4 per cent (Anon. 1997). T-Cell lymphomas are more common in Asia and there is a high incidence of nasal-type natural killer (NK)/T-cell lymphomas in Asian races. In parts of Japan and the Caribbean, the increased incidence of adult T-cell leukaemia/lymphoma is related to the high prevalence of infection by the human T-cell leukaemia/lymphoma virus 1(HTLV-1).

For a number of reasons, the classification of tumours derived from postthymic or mature T-cells is less satisfactory than the classification of B-cell neoplasms. With the exception of diffuse large B-cell lymphoma, which remains a heterogeneous group, the current World Health Organisation (WHO) classification of B-cell lymphomas reflects reasonably well their histogenesis and provides a guide to treatment. By contrast, neoplastic T-cells show marked morphological variation. They may be difficult to characterize because of variable or aberrant expression of the T-cell antigens, and their relationship to the normal sequence of T-cell maturation and differentiation is far from clear. Some tumours exhibit combined features of T-cells and the closely related natural killer (NK) cells and it is usual to consider T-cell and NK-cell neoplasms together.

Classifications of T-cell lymphomas have been an uncomfortable mix of purely descriptive terms and fairly well-defined entities. The Working Formulation made no attempt to separate lymphomas according to phenotype, and T-cell lymphomas were hidden in descriptive terminology designed primarily for B-cell tumours. The Kiel classification improved on this by recognizing T-cell neoplasms and separating them into low-grade and high-grade categories. The least satisfactory area concerned nodal T-cell lymphomas. With the exception of anaplastic large cell lymphoma and angioimmunoblastic lymphoma, both of which are now fairly well characterized, node-based peripheral T-cell lymphomas remained a poorly defined group, which could not be subclassified with any degree of consistency.

The REAL classification (Harris et al. 1994) and, most recently, the WHO classification (Jaffe et al. 2001) attempted an objective reassessment and accepted only those entities that can be reliably distinguished on clinical, pathological or genetic grounds. They recognize a number of well-defined T-cell neoplasms, some of which are primarily extranodal or leukaemic, and they leave largely intact a group of node-based peripheral T-cell lymphomas under the umbrella term 'unspecified', on the basis that further subclassification is subject to considerable interobserver variation and has little clinical validity. Developments in molecular techniques and clinicopathological studies of large series of cases may help to identify further defined entities within this group.

Leukaemias and extranodal lymphomas fall outside the scope of a book concerned with lymph node pathology; however, some show secondary involvement of lymph nodes and it is important, therefore, to recognize their features. The modification of the WHO

BOX 6.1: Lymph node involvement by T-cell lymphomas

T-CELL LYMPHOMAS WITH PRIMARY NODAL INVOLVEMENT
Angioimmunoblastic T-cell lymphoma
Anaplastic large cell lymphoma
Peripheral T-cell lymphoma – unspecified

T-CELL LEUKAEMIA/LYMPHOMAS WITH NODAL INVOLVEMENT
Precursor T-lymphoblastic leukaemia/lymphoma (see page 52)
Adult T-cell leukaemia/lymphoma
T-Cell prolymphocytic leukaemia

EXTRANODAL T-CELL LYMPHOMAS WITH SECONDARY NODAL INVOLVEMENT
Enteropathy-type T-cell lymphoma

Primary cutaneous CD30+ T-cell anaplastic large cell lymphoma
Mycosis fungoides/Sézary syndrome

EXTRANODAL LYMPHOMAS WITH EARLY NODAL INVOLVEMENT
Blastic NK-cell lymphoma

EXTRANODAL T-CELL LYMPHOMAS RARELY SHOWING NODAL INVOLVEMENT
Extranodal NK/T-cell lymphoma, nasal type
Hepatosplenic T-cell lymphoma
Subcutaneous panniculitis-like T-cell lymphoma

T-CELL LEUKAEMIAS
T-Cell large granular lymphocytic leukaemia
Aggressive NK-cell leukaemia

---

classification shown in Box 6.1 indicates which tumours are primarily nodal and which involve nodes secondarily.

ANGIOIMMUNOBLASTIC LYMPHOMA

In the mid-1970s, the first descriptions of angioimmunoblastic lymphoma (AILT) as 'immunoblastic lymphadenopathy' or 'angioimmunoblastic lymphadenopathy with dysproteinaemia' regarded it as an essentially reactive systemic process but recognized that it was at least premalignant and carried a poor prognosis, with a proportion of patients developing frank lymphoma. Until that time, it seems likely that most cases were diagnosed as Hodgkin lymphoma or an unspecified reactive process. Not until monoclonal T-cell populations could be demonstrated by molecular techniques did it become clear that, at least in the majority of cases, AILT is a T-cell neoplasm from the outset (Dogan 2003).

Like most lymphomas, the aetiology of AILT is unknown. In early series, many of the patients had a history of medication, particularly with antibiotics, but it is likely that these were given because systemic symptoms in the early stages of the disease can mimic an infectious process. Search for a viral cause has shown an interesting association with the Epstein–Barr virus (EBV), which is further discussed below, but no other convincing associations.

AILT accounts for about 15–20 per cent of T-cell lymphomas and 1–2 per cent of all non-Hodgkin lymphomas. Most patients are aged between 50 and 70 years, with a median age of 59–64 years and equal sex incidence. They typically present with systemic symptoms, generalized lymphadenopathy and hepatosplenomegaly. Some also have a skin rash with pruritis. Other features include ascites, pleural effusions and arthritis. Investigations show a polyclonal hypergammaglobulinaemia, elevated erythrocyte sedimentation rate (ESR) and lactate dehydrogenase (LDH), and anaemia, often of Coombs-positive autoimmune type. Other autoantibodies, such as rheumatoid factor, thyroid autoantibodies and antismooth muscle antibodies may be present.

Despite intensive chemotherapy, the prognosis remains poor, with a 5-year survival of only 20–30 per cent. This is partly due to the immune deficiency associated with the disease and many patients develop fatal infectious complications.

HISTOLOGY

Primary diagnosis of AILT usually depends on lymph node biopsy. Biopsies from involved extranodal sites, such as skin, spleen, liver, bone marrow and lung, are less reliable because the diagnosis is dependent on a combination of architectural and cytological features.

The features originally used to define angioimmunoblastic lymphadenopathy were the presence of arborizing blood vessels surrounded by amorphous periodic acid–Schiff (PAS)-positive material and a polymorphic infiltrate, including plasma cells, histiocytes, neutrophils and eosinophils. The presence of scattered large, blast-like cells, some of which resembled Hodgkin/Reed–Sternberg (RS) cells, was also identified as a consistent feature. Early descriptions did not stress the presence of clear cells but it is now recognized that these represent the malignant population. These are medium to large cells with clear cytoplasm that occur singly and in clusters. They vary in prominence and degree of atypia and tend to occur around the proliferating vessels. The majority of AILT biopsies also include hypocellular, eosinophilic areas corresponding to areas of burnt-out follicles in which there is dendritic cell proliferation. While this remains a useful feature, it is now recognized that cases with hyperplastic follicles may occur (Ree *et al.* 1998).

The arborizing high endothelial vessels are highlighted in sections stained for reticulin and in PAS-stained sections in which the vessels are seen to be surrounded by a thick layer of PAS-positive basement membrane material. The polymorphic infiltrate effaces the normal lymph node structure and often extends into the perinodal tissues, characteristically leaving a gaping subcapsular sinus (Ottavianni *et al.* 2004).

IMMUNOHISTOCHEMISTRY

The majority of the cells in the infiltrate express the T-cell markers, CD3 and CD5. Most are also CD4 positive with a minor population of CD8-positive cells. Residual B-cell areas are identified by CD20 and CD79a, often as small irregular aggregates at the periphery of the node. Many of the large blasts scattered throughout the node are also identified as B-cells. The markers for follicular dendritic cells, CD21, CD23 and CD35, show a very distinctive proliferation of these cells, producing an expanded dendritic meshwork corresponding to the eosinophilic material seen in haematoxylin and eosin (H&E) stains (Jones *et al.* 1998).

A recently described and helpful feature of the AILT is the expression of CD10 and, less consistently, BCL-6, antigens usually associated with follicle centre B-cells. These stain a population of CD4+ T-cells, corresponding to the medium-sized clear cells seen in relation to the vessels and the dendritic cell networks. Single cell microdissection studies of these cells indicate that they are monoclonal and represent the neoplastic population

(Attygale *et al.* 2002). However, the number of CD10+ cells in involved nodes varies considerably and they may be difficult to appreciate. Similar CD10+ cells may also be identified in extranodal deposits, again related to a follicular dendritic cell network (Attygale *et al.* 2004).

The large B-blasts seen in AILT are often CD30 positive and, in many cases, can be shown to be EBV positive.

GENETICS

Southern blotting techniques and the polymerase chain reaction (PCR) have established the presence of clonal rearrangement of T-cell receptor genes in AILT. However, immunoglobulin gene rearrangement may also be identified in a significant number of cases. It has been suggested that these B-cell clones are related to the proliferation of EBV-driven cells, made possible by the immunodeficiency associated with AILT, a situation analogous to post-transplant lymphoproliferative disease.

Cytogenetic studies reveal both clonal and non-clonal abnormalities, the most consistent being trisomy 3, trisomy 5 and an additional X chromosome.

DIFFERENTIAL DIAGNOSIS

When there is complete effacement of the node, it is unlikely that AILT can be mistaken for reactive lymphadenopathy. However, in those cases where reactive B-follicles are preserved, the distinction from a reactive process, such as a florid viral infection, may be difficult. Consideration of the clinical setting should alert the pathologist to the possibility of AILT. If necessary, molecular studies with PCR may be used to establish clonality.

The presence of CD30-positive, Reed–Sternberg-like cells may suggest classical Hodgkin lymphoma of mixed

---

▲ BOX 6.2: Angioimmunoblastic lymphoma: clinical features

- ▲ Systemic symptoms
- ▲ Widespread lymphadenopathy and hepatosplenomegaly
- ▲ Rash
- ▲ Hypergammaglobulinaemia
- ▲ Haemolytic anaemia
- ▲ Other autoantibodies

● BOX 6.3: Angioimmunoblastic lymphoma: morphology

- Complete or partial effacement of node
- Extension into perinodal tissues, often leaving subcapsular sinus patent
- Mixed population of reactive and neoplastic cells
- Scattered B-blasts – Epstein–Barr virus (EBV) positive
- Prominent, branching high-endothelial venules surrounded by periodic acid–Schiff (PAS)-positive basement membrane
- Expanded follicular dendritic cell network
- Clusters of medium sized T-cells with clear cytoplasm.

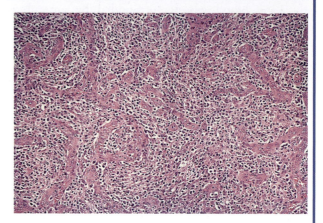

FIGURE 6.3 The characteristic vascular proliferation in angioimmunoblastic lymphoma is due to 'arborizing' postcapillary or high-endothelial venules.

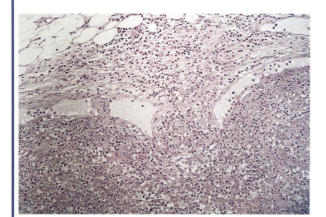

FIGURE 6.1 Angioimmunoblastic lymphoma. Even when the infiltrate extends beyond the capsule of the node into surrounding tissue, there is a tendency for the peripheral sinus to remain widely patent.

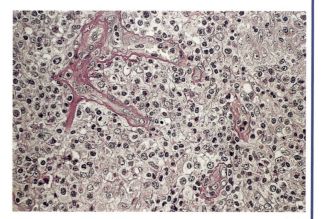

FIGURE 6.4 Angioimmunoblastic lymphoma. The vessels are well seen in periodic acid–Schiff stains owing to staining of the basement membranes.

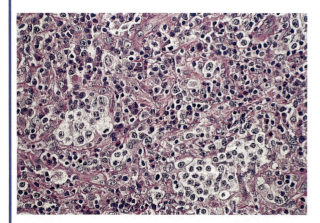

FIGURE 6.2 The typical polymorphous infiltrate in angioimmunoblastic lymphoma includes plasma cells, large blasts, eosinophils and clear cells.

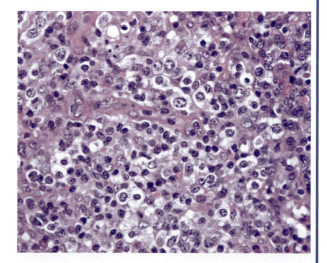

FIGURE 6.5 Clear cells. The neoplastic cells in angio-immunoblastic lymphoma tend to cluster around vessels, and have clear cytoplasm with nuclei of intermediate size and variable pleomorphism.

◆ **BOX 6.4: Angioimmunoblastic lymphoma: immunohistochemistry**

- CD3, CD5, CD4-positive T-cells, often CD10 positive
- Residual B-cell areas (CD20 and CD79a positive) pushed to periphery of node
- CD20, CD79a-positive blasts, often CD30 positive

- B-blasts may express Epstein–Barr virus (EBV)-encoded RNAs (EBERs) and EBV antigens
- Expanded network of dendritic cells demonstrated by CD21, CD23, CD35.

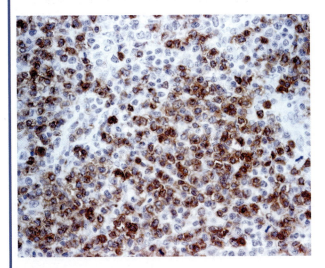

FIGURE 6.6 Angioimmunoblastic lymphoma. Many of the clear cells express CD10.

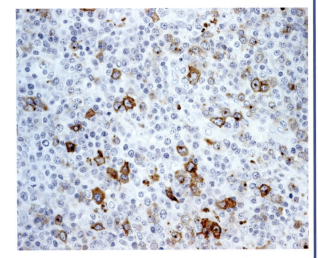

FIGURE 6.8 Angioimmunoblastic lymphoma: CD30. Scattered large blasts express B-cell markers and are frequently CD30 positive.

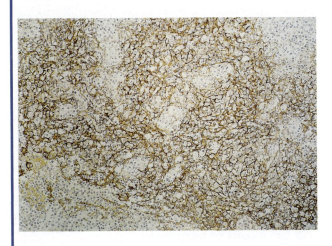

FIGURE 6.7 Angioimmunoblastic lymphoma: CD21. Both CD21 and CD23 can be used to demonstrate the complex network of follicular dendritic cells associated with the vascular proliferation.

cellularity type. These RS-like cells usually lack typical morphological features, particularly inclusion-like nucleoli, and are CD15 negative. Unlike Hodgkin cells, they consistently express CD45 and the B-cell markers CD20 and CD79a. Attention to the background will demonstrate the other features of AILT.

Other T-cell lymphomas may have a similar polymorphic population to AILT but lack some of the typical features, particularly CD10-positive T-cells. Whether these should be grouped with AILT is debatable and not at present of great clinical relevance. The presence of widespread disease and systemic symptoms should be taken into consideration if the histological appearances are equivocal.

Scattered, large, blast-like B-cells in a mixed background with large numbers of T-cells may suggest large B-cell lymphoma of T-cell-rich or T-cell histiocyte-rich type. The typical vascular pattern, the mix and distribution of the cells, and the pattern of the follicular dendritic network should help make the distinction from AILT.

ANAPLASTIC LARGE CELL LYMPHOMA

Anaplastic large cell lymphoma (ALCL) was first described as a specific entity by Stein and his colleagues in 1985 (Stein *et al.* 1985, 2000, Jaffe 2001). This followed identification of the antigen that was originally called Ki-1 but subsequently designated CD30, a 120-kDa transmembrane cytokine receptor of the tumour necrosis factor (TNF) receptor family. The CD30 antigen is expressed on the Hodgkin/Reed–Sternberg (H/RS) cells of classic Hodgkin lymphoma and in normal lymph nodes by activated lymphoid blasts typically scattered around reactive B-cell follicles. The large tumour cells of ALCL uniformly and strongly express CD30 on the cell membrane and in the Golgi region. It is often weakly expressed or not expressed on the small cells of the small cell and lymphohistiocytic variants of ALCL, although it is more consistently positive on the large cells found in such tumours.

It was subsequently found that many examples of ALCL had a t(2;5) chromosomal translocation, causing the NPM (nucleophosmin) gene located on 5q35 to fuse with a gene on 2p23 encoding the tyrosine kinase receptor, anaplastic lymphoma kinase (ALK).

Anaplastic large cell lymphoma constitutes 2 per cent of all lymphomas, but forms 10 per cent or more of childhood lymphomas. ALK-positive cases have a bimodal age distribution with the major peak in the second decade and a small peak in later life. It is more common in males, particularly in the younger age group. Most patients have advanced disease with systemic symptoms at the time of presentation. The majority have lymphadenopathy but extranodal disease is frequent and, in a small number of patients, ALCL is exclusively extranodal. Skin, bone, soft tissues, bone marrow, lung and liver are the most frequently involved sites. Leukaemic peripheral blood involvement is uncommon and is an indicator of poor prognosis (Onciu *et al.* 2003).

ALK-negative tumours occur in an older age group, have a lower male to female ratio and tend to present at an earlier stage. Untreated ALCL pursues an aggressive course but patients with ALK-positive tumours have a good response to treatment with excellent (>75 per cent) overall survival. ALK-negative tumours behave similarly to other types of peripheral T-cell lymphoma with a relatively poor prognosis.

▲ BOX 6.5: Anaplastic large cell lymphoma: clinical features

- ▲ Most common in young people with peak in second decade
- ▲ Male predominance
- ▲ Widespread disease with B symptoms, often extranodal
- ▲ ALK+ tumours have good prognosis
- ▲ ALK− tumours behave as T-cell lymphoma, unspecified.

HISTOLOGY

The histology of ALCL is variable but all variants contain at least occasional hallmark cells. These are large cells with reniform or horseshoe nuclei, and abundant eosinophilic or amphophilic cytoplasm. The nuclei usually contain several nucleoli that may appear basophilic or eosinophilic. Multinucleated cells in which the nuclei form a wreath-like circle are sometimes seen. Binucleate forms may resemble RS cells, although they do not usually show the prominent eosinophilic nucleoli of the latter. Cells of ALCL often appear cohesive and, in lymph node biopsies, may be seen within preserved sinuses, giving an appearance suggestive of metastatic carcinoma or melanoma. ALCL cells also have a propensity to accumulate around blood vessels.

ALCL common variant

This variant accounts for 70–80 per cent of cases. The tumour cells are large and have abundant cytoplasm. The nuclear morphology varies from pleomorphic to predominantly rounded and monomorphic. Hallmark cells can usually be identified.

ALCL lymphohistiocytic variant

This variant accounts for approximately 10 per cent of cases. Since histiocytes are the dominant cell and may obscure the neoplastic cells, this subtype needs to be recognized. The tumour cells that may be relatively small are highlighted by immunostaining for CD30 or ALK, and may be clustered around blood vessels. The non-neoplastic histiocytes may show erythrophagocytosis.

ALCL small cell variant

This is an uncommon variant that may easily be mistaken for peripheral T-cell lymphoma – unspecified. The small to medium neoplastic cells have irregular nuclei. Hallmark cells are often clustered around blood vessels and are highlighted by staining for CD30, which is expressed more strongly on these cells than on the small cells.

Other variants

In addition to the above variants recognized in the WHO classification, other histological patterns have been reported. A hypocellular variant associated with a myxoid stroma mimicking an inflammatory process has been reported (Cheuk *et al.* 2000). Spindle cell sarcomatoid, signet ring and giant-cell-rich subtypes have also been reported (Benharroch et al. 1998). Different subtypes may be seen in the same patient at different sites and at different times.

IMMUNOHISTOCHEMISTRY

In the classical variant of ALCL, CD30 is strongly and uniformly expressed on the cell membrane and in the Golgi region. CD30 expression in the small cell variant may be weaker or more variable, with strongest expression on perivascular large cells. ALK protein is expressed in 60–90 per cent of tumours. The commonest pattern of expression, associated with t(2;5), shows positive nuclear and cytoplasmic staining. Other less common translocations give rise to membrane or cytoplasmic staining. Epithelial membrane antigen (EMA) expression is seen in all ALK-positive tumours but is less commonly expressed in ALK-negative cases. CD45 and CD45RO are variably expressed in ALCL. Expression of T-cell antigens is variable, but ALCL generally lacks expression of T-cell receptor molecules or molecules of proximal T-cell receptor signalling (Bonzheim *et al.* 2004). Most ALCL express one or more T-cell markers, but some are of the 'null cell' phenotype. CD4 is most often positive, CD3 is expressed by less than 25 per cent of tumours, CD5 and CD7 are frequently

---

● **BOX 6.6: Anaplastic large cell lymphoma: morphology**

- May have sinusoidal growth pattern with cohesive cells
- Hallmark cells found in all types but typical of 'common' type

- Variants include small cell, lymphohistiocytic, giant cell, monomorphic and sarcomatoid
- Pattern may be mixed in same site or different nodes.

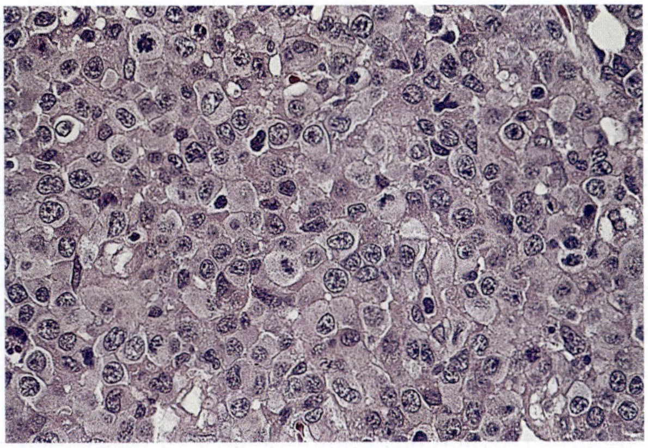

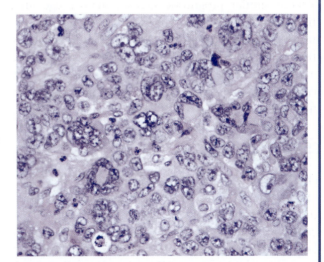

FIGURE 6.9 In the 'common' variant of anaplastic large cell lymphoma, cells show the features of large blasts, often with fairly abundant cytoplasm and forming cohesive sheets. Scattered hallmark cells are present.

FIGURE 6.10 Anaplastic large cell lymphoma. Other examples show more marked pleomorphism with atypical mitoses. Nuclei are open and lobated, and include the hallmark cells, in which the lobes form horseshoe or ring shapes.

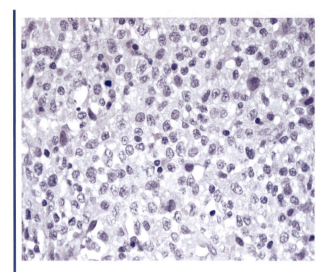

FIGURE 6.11 In this small cell variant of anaplastic large cell lymphoma, nuclei are smaller and irregular and many lack prominent nucleoli.

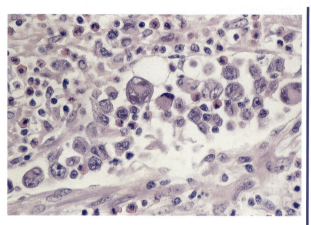

FIGURE 6.12 Anaplastic large cell lymphoma. A sinus pattern of spread is typical of early nodal involvement.

negative, and CD8 is usually negative. Most tumours are positive for the cytotoxic granule markers, TIA-1, granzyme and perforin, and some express CD56.

ALK-negative anaplastic large cell lymphoma

Anaplastic lymphoma kinase-negative ALCL is a more heterogeneous entity than the ALK-positive neoplasm. Its distinction from other types of peripheral T-cell lymphoma of either 'unspecified' or angioimmunoblastic type is of less clinical importance because similar prognostic factors, mainly age and International Prognostic Index (IPI), apply. In contrast to ALK-positive tumours, ALK-negative tumours show weak expression of EMA and cytotoxic granule markers. By definition, most have a common-type morphology but some giant cell rich variants are included in this category.

GENETICS

The 2;5 translocation causes the NPM gene located at 5q35 to fuse with a gene at 2p23 encoding the tyrosine kinase receptor anaplastic lymphoma kinase. Transcription of the NPM-ALK hybrid gene results in production of NPM-ALK or p80. The presence of nuclear staining in addition to cytoplasmic staining is explained by the formation of dimers between NPM-ALK and wild-type nucleophosmin, which provides a nuclear signal and allows the dimer to enter the nucleus. The t(1;2) translocation occurs in about 10–20 per cent of

ALK + ALCL, leading to fusion of the ALK gene with the tropomysin 3 (TPM3) gene, and results in cytoplasmic and cell membrane staining. Less common translocations, t(2;3), Inv2, t(2;17), produce only cytoplasmic staining.

Despite the very variable expression of T-cell antigens, it is possible by PCR to demonstrate that the majority (90 per cent) of ALCL show clonal rearrangement of the T-cell receptor (TCR) genes.

DIFFERENTIAL DIAGNOSIS

Metastatic carcinoma and melanoma are readily excluded by staining for cytokeratins, S100 and HMB45.

Pleomorphic diffuse large B-cell lymphomas may express CD30, particularly on the more atypical cells. These tumours otherwise have the phenotype of diffuse large B-cell lymphoma (DLBCL) and should not be categorized as ALCL. Rare DLBCL have the morphology of ALCL and uniformly express CD30 but not ALK. They express B-cell lineage markers and, in the WHO classification, are categorized as a subset of DLBCL. The exception is a rare form of large B-cell lymphoma, which has immunoblastic or plasmablastic morphology, and expresses ALK but not CD30 (see Chapter 5; Delsol *et al.* 1997, Adam *et al.* 2003, Morris 2003). Other tumours in which ALK expression has been identified include inflammatory myofibroblastic tumours and some glioblastomas.

The distinction between ALCL and classical Hodgkin lymphoma has important implications for treatment

◆ BOX 6.7: Anaplastic large cell lymphoma: immunophenotype

- CD30 expression essential
- Anaplastic lymphoma kinase (ALK) expression provides important division into prognostic groups
- Epithelial membrane antigen (EMA) typically positive in ALK+ tumours
- CD3, CD5, CD7, CD8 usually negative, CD4 more often positive
- T-Cell intracellular antigen (TIA)-1, granzyme, perforin usually positive in ALK+ tumours
- CD56 often positive.

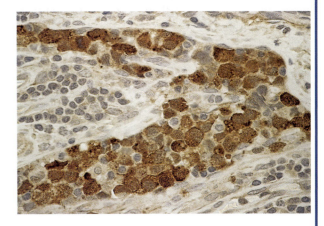

FIGURE 6.14 Anaplastic large cell lymphoma. Anaplastic lymphoma kinase (ALK) staining is both nuclear and cytoplasmic when the ALK/NPM (p80) translocation is present.

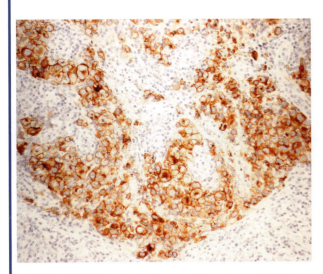

FIGURE 6.13 Anaplastic large cell lymphoma. CD30 staining typically shows membrane and Golgi positivity similar to that seen in Hodgkin lymphoma. CD30 is useful in identifying cells in the sinuses.

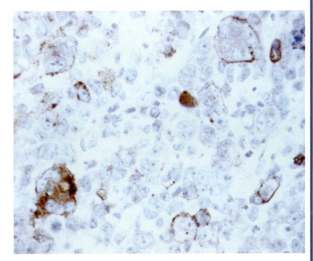

FIGURE 6.15 Expression of epithelial membrane antigen by anaplastic large cell lymphoma is variable and usually associated with anaplastic lymphoma kinase-positive tumours. The staining pattern is similar to CD30 with membrane and Golgi positivity, but tends to be more granular.

and prognosis, and may be difficult. This applies particularly to those cases that lack expression of both ALK and CD15 and contain RS-like or multinucleate cells. By giving careful consideration to the expanded immunophenotype (Table 6.1), and, if necessary, to molecular techniques, it should possible to make the distinction. The concept of a borderline group of 'ALCL–Hodgkin-like' lymphoma has been reassessed and the term is not retained in the WHO classification. The majority of such cases are eventually classified as Hodgkin lymphoma. However, there remain occasional 'grey zone' lymphomas that continue to cause problems in classification. These include tumours with Hodgkin-like cells expressing both CD30 and CD15, in which one or more of the T-cell markers or the cytotoxic granule markers are positive and B-cell markers are negative. Expression of EBV-related antigens may be helpful in these cases as ALCL is usually negative.

Cutaneous lesions of CD30+ lymphoma are seen in both primary cutaneous CD30+ anaplastic large cell

Table 6.1: Differential diagnosis of anaplastic large cell lymphoma: immunophenotype

	ALK+ ANAPLASTIC LARGE CELL LYMPHOMA	ALK− ANAPLASTIC LARGE CELL LYMPHOMA	CLASSICAL HODGKIN LYMPHOMA H/RS CELLS	DIFFUSE LARGE B-CELL LYMPHOMA	ALK+ DIFFUSE LARGE B-CELL LYMPHOMA
CD30	Positive membrane and Golgi	Positive membrane and Golgi	Positive membrane and Golgi	Variably positive; may show anaplastic morphology	Negative
ALK	Positive; usually nuclear and cytoplasmic	Negative	Negative	Negative	Positive; granular cytoplasmic and Golgi
CD20	Negative	Negative	Variable c. 20 per cent weakly positive	Positive	Negative
T-cell antigens	Variable; CD3, 4, 5 or 'null'	Variable CD3, 4, 5 or 'null'	Rarely weakly positive	Negative	Negative
EMA	Positive membrane and Golgi	Variable and weak	Negative	Negative	Positive membrane, variable Golgi
CD45	Positive	Variable and weak	Negative	Positive	Positive
CD15	Negative	Negative	Positive in c. 75 per cent	Negative	Negative
Cytotoxic T-cell markers	Positive (TIA-1, granzyme, perforin)	Variable and weak	Usually negative	Negative	Negative

ALK, anaplastic lymphoma kinase; EMA, epithelial membrane antigen; H/RS, Hodgkin/Reed–Sternberg; TIA, T-cell intracellular antigen.

BOX 6.8: Tumours with CD30 anaplastic large cell morphology

- ALK+ anaplastic large cell lymphoma;
- ALK− anaplastic large cell lymphoma;
- anaplastic variants of diffuse large B-cell lymphoma;
- primary cutaneous anaplastic large cell lymphoma;
- intestinal T-cell lymphoma (enteropathy-associated T-cell lymphoma) (see page 108);
- adult T-cell lymphoma/leukaemia (see page 104);
- peripheral T-cell lymphoma – unspecified (see page 101).

lymphoma of T-cell type (including lymphomatoid papulosis) or cutaneous manifestations of systemic ALCL. ALK expression is not a feature of the former and EMA is often negative. The presence of these markers implies systemic disease with a significantly better response to treatment and prognosis.

PERIPHERAL T-CELL LYMPHOMA – UNSPECIFIED

In some respects, peripheral T-cell lymphoma, unspecified (PTLU) is a diagnosis of exclusion. The term covers the 50 per cent or so of peripheral T-cell lymphomas that do not fall into any of the other, better defined categories and is, therefore, a heterogeneous group with very variable morphological features. Clinically, it is one of the more aggressive forms of non-Hodgkin lymphoma. It is primarily a disease of adults with an equal sex ratio. Most patients have systemic symptoms and extranodal disease is frequent. Bone marrow, liver, spleen and skin are frequently involved sites and there may be a leukaemic phase with peripheral blood involvement. Less frequent manifestations are due to abnormal production of cytokines and include eosinophilia and haemophagocytic syndrome (Ascani et al. 1997).

HISTOLOGY

In most cases, involved lymph nodes are diffusely infiltrated with complete effacement of normal nodal structure. The infiltrate may be monomorphic, consisting almost entirely of neoplastic cells, or polymorphic, with a mixed background of small lymphocytes, eosinophils, plasma cells and histiocytes. As in angioimmunoblastic T-cell lymphoma, vessels may be prominent. Sometimes the pattern may be more clearly interfollicular with preservation of normal or even hyperplastic follicles. It is likely that this so-called *T-zone variant* represents an earlier stage in node involvement rather than a separate entity (Suchi et al. 1987).

The malignant cells show a range of morphological features and sizes. In the majority of tumours, nuclei are intermediate or large when compared with histiocyte nuclei. They frequently show some degree of irregularity or folding and tend to be hyperchromatic with indistinct nucleoli. In other examples, they may be vesicular with prominent nucleoli and resemble centroblasts or immunoblasts. The cytoplasm may be pale or clear with distinct cell borders and a perifollicular

pattern is described in which the appearances resemble nodal marginal zone lymphoma (Rudiger et al. 2000). Markedly pleomorphic cells with polylobated nuclei may resemble those seen in anaplastic large cell lymphoma and, if these are CD30-positive, the distinction from ALK-ALCL becomes blurred.

The background, non-neoplastic cell population may include clusters of epithelioid histiocytes. In the Kiel classification, such tumours were designated *lymphoepithelioid T-cell lymphoma* [Lennert lymphoma (Suchi et al. 1987)]. This is a descriptive term that has not been shown to have clinical implications and it is doubtful whether it should be regarded as a distinct entity. Epithelioid histiocytes are not infrequent in peripheral T-cell lymphomas and there is no guide as to how many are needed for a diagnosis of lymphoepithelioid cell lymphoma. Abundant histiocytes and other reactive background cells may, however, obscure the malignant cell population and make diagnosis more difficult.

The WHO classification resists the temptation to attempt further subclassification of PTLU on purely descriptive grounds but previous classifications have used cell size as the criterion (Jaffe et al. 2001). The REAL classification, for example, provisionally divided tumours into those with medium-sized cells, mixed medium and large cells, and large cells (Harris et al. 1994). These subdivisions are subjective and do not at present appear to have clinical validity. Peripheral T-cell lymphomas in general have a poor 5-year survival, with age and International Prognostic Index being the main prognostic factors.

IMMUNOHISTOCHEMISTRY

In paraffin sections, using the commonly available T-cell markers, CD3, CD4, CD5, CD7, CD8, CD43 and CD45RO, a variety of T-cell phenotypes can be identified and aberrant phenotypes are common. Most tumours express CD3, but CD5 and CD7 are frequently lost. CD4 and CD8 expression is also very variable and cells may express one, both or neither antigen. It is suggested that lymphoepithelioid T-cell lymphoma more often expresses CD8 and may be derived from cytotoxic T-cells (Geissinger et al. 2004). CD30 is frequently positive, particularly in large cell variants. It is unusual to find expression of the cytotoxic granule markers and CD56 in nodal lymphomas.

Occasionally, scattered large cells resemble H/RS cells and may have an identical immunophenotype, expressing CD20, CD30 and even occasionally CD15. EBV-related antigens are also expressed and this may represent expansion of EBV-infected clones related to the immunodeficiency associated with the T-cell lymphoma (Quintanilla-Martinez *et al.* 1999).

GENETICS

Proof of clonality in T-cell proliferations depends on molecular techniques and PCR can be used to demonstrate clonal rearrangement of the T-cell receptor genes. Peripheral T-cell lymphomas show a wide range of cytogenetic abnormalities but no consistent clonal abnormality has been identified.

DIFFERENTIAL DIAGNOSIS

In those tumours with a polymorphic background of non-neoplastic cells, particularly where follicles are preserved ('T-zone lymphoma'), it may be difficult to appreciate that the atypical cells are neoplastic T-cells rather than the activated blasts seen in a variety of reactive conditions. However, they tend to form a more clearly atypical population and immunohistochemistry reveals their T-cell phenotype. If epithelioid histiocytes are prominent, other granulomatous conditions should be considered. Toxoplasmosis is rarely a consideration because the architecture is not obscured and prominent reactive B-cell follicles are characteristic of this condition. The well-defined epithelioid and giant cell granulomas seen in sarcoidosis and granulomatous infections are rare in T-cell lymphoma, but are an occasional feature and may even show some degree of central necrosis.

In some peripheral T-cell lymphomas, large pleomorphic cells may resemble Hodgkin or RS cells. When they are scattered in a mixed background that includes eosinophils, plasma cells and histiocytes, classical Hodgkin lymphoma becomes the major differential diagnosis. CD30 is unreliable in making the distinction as many T-cell lymphomas express this antigen to a variable extent. CD15 is helpful in identifying Hodgkin lymphoma if it is positive. T-cell and B-cell markers are clearly useful: Hodgkin cells only rarely express T-cell antigens and, in about 30 per cent of cases, weak expression of CD20 is seen.

Although the distinction between PTLU and diffuse large B-cell lymphoma may not be immediately clear on routinely stained sections, it should present no problem once the basic immunohistochemical profile is completed. T-cell, histiocyte-rich, B-cell lymphoma may be more difficult to distinguish. The large atypical B-cells are usually clearly seen against the background of small T-lymphocytes and histiocytes, but initial impressions, particularly on small and inadequate biopsies, may suggest a neoplastic T-cell population.

Although anaplastic large cell lymphoma and angioimmunoblastic lymphoma are now well-defined entities, both show some overlap with PTLU. Anaplastic large cell lymphoma should be considered if the tumour cells are large and pleomorphic with multilobated nuclei, particularly if they express CD30. If ALK is negative, staining for EMA and the cytotoxic granule markers rarely help to decide whether the tumour should be categorized as ALK− anaplastic large cell lymphoma. To some extent this may be academic, as the natural history and prognosis of ALK− tumours do not differ from T-cell lymphoma – unspecified. Similarly, it makes very little difference at present to patient management or survival if tumours showing only some of the features of angioimmunoblastic lymphoma are classified as such or as PTLU. In general, those with large numbers of clearly atypical cells are more suitably classified as the latter.

▲ **BOX 6.9: Peripheral T-cell lymphoma – unspecified: clinical features**

- ▲ Uncommon lymphomas with geographical and racial variations
- ▲ Usually adults with equal sex ratio
- ▲ Widespread disease and systemic symptoms frequent
- ▲ Poor response to treatment and low 5-year survival

● **BOX 6.10: Peripheral T-cell lymphoma – unspecified: morphology**

- Infiltrate monomorphic or polymorphic
- Wide variation in cell size, typically medium to large
- Wide variation in nuclear morphology
- Epithelioid cell clusters often present.

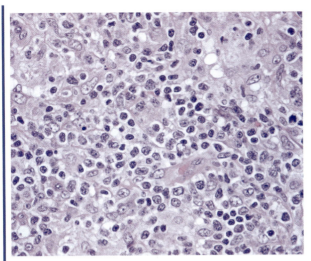

FIGURE 6.16 The infiltrate in peripheral T-cell lymphoma – unspecified is frequently polymorphous with neoplastic cells of varying sizes with irregular nuclei. In this example, some have clear cytoplasm similar to those seen in angioimmunoblastic lymphoma.

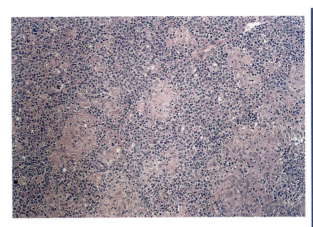

FIGURE 6.17 The so-called Lennert lymphoma is a peripheral T-cell lymphoma – unspecified in which cohesive clusters of epithelioid histiocytes are prominent.

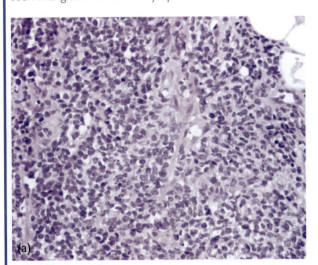

(a)

FIGURE 6.18 Peripheral T-cell lymphoma – unspecified: intermediate cell morphology. (a) The tumour cells have irregular, small to medium-sized, uniformly hyperchromatic nuclei.

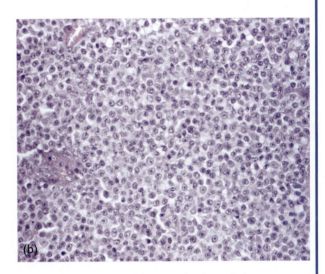

(b)

FIGURE 6.18 (b) In this example, the cells have rounded, fairly uniform nuclei, most a with a single prominent nucleolus.

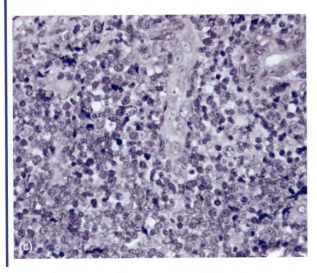

(c)

FIGURE 6.18 (c) The neoplastic cells show more variation in size with occasional large blasts. For comparison the majority are slightly smaller than the endothelial cells.

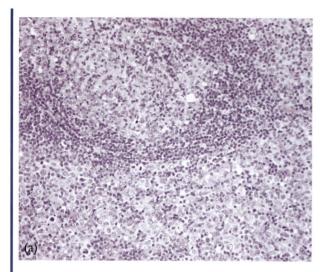

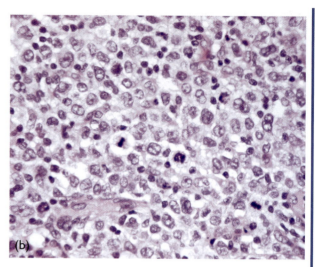

FIGURE 6.19 Peripheral T-cell lymphoma – unspecified: large cell morphology. (a) Infiltration of the T-zone may lead to sparing of the B-cell follicles, seen here in a large cell variant.

FIGURE 6.19 (b) In this example, cells have large, open, irregular, folded nuclei, one or more nucleoli and abundant pale or clear cytoplasm.

◆ **BOX 6.11: Peripheral T-cell lymphoma – unspecified: immunohistochemistry**

- Aberrant T-cell phenotypes common
- CD3 usually positive
- CD5 and CD7 often lost
- CD4, CD8 very variable
- CD56 and cytotoxic granule markers unusual
- CD30 variably positive

ADULT T-CELL LEUKAEMIA/LYMPHOMA

Adult T-cell leukaemia/lymphoma (ATLL) is causally related to infection with the retrovirus, human T-cell leukaemia virus type 1 (HTLV-1). Sporadic cases do occur but the disease is concentrated in those areas where the virus is endemic. In parts of Japan, particularly on the island of Kyushu, where about 10 per cent of the population are seropositive, the virus is widespread and may be transmitted through blood and blood products, by breast milk from mother to child, or between sexual partners. Clusters of disease also occur in parts of West Africa, in Black patients from the Caribbean and the south-eastern USA, and in Black communities in cities such as New York. In New York and New Orleans, between 10 and 25 per cent of

intravenous drug abusers are seropositive for HTLV-1. Neoplastic transformation does not depend only on the presence of the virus (only about one in 1000 seropositive individuals develop ATTL) but is presumed to follow additional oncogenic events. The virus infects the CD4+ (helper) T-cells and a definitive diagnosis can be made by demonstrating the HTLV-1 proviral DNA in the tumour cell DNA by PCR.

Adult T-cell leukaemia/lymphoma is a systemic disease and the majority of patients present with Stage IV disease, with widespread lymph node involvement and circulating atypical cells in the peripheral blood. About half of the patients also have skin involvement, hepatosplenomegaly is frequently present and the bone marrow is involved in about 60 per cent. In Japanese patients, 'smouldering' or chronic forms of the disease are described in which circulating cells are uncommon. In the lymphomatous variant, lymphadenopathy is more prominent and circulating tumour cells are not seen. In the acute and lymphomatous types, therapy is largely ineffective and the prognosis is poor (Shimoyama 1991).

One of the most characteristic features of ATLL is hypercalcaemia, often accompanied by lytic bone lesions. Bone biopsy shows increased osteoclastic activity and this may lead to a diagnosis of hyperparathyroidism. Blood eosinophilia is present in some cases.

The diagnosis of ATLL is usually made on the presence of the characteristic cells in the peripheral blood. These are pleomorphic and show considerable variation in size. Nuclear lobation is the most typical feature, giving rise to the term 'flower cells'.

HISTOLOGY

Lymph node biopsy from patients with acute and lymphomatous forms of the disease shows diffuse infiltration and apparent loss of architecture. However, reticulin stains may demonstrate retention of the underlying structure of the node and sinuses may be seen. Cell size is very variable. In some cases, small cells predominate or there is a mixture of small and large cells. In the majority of cases, they are intermediate to large with prominent nucleoli and clumped chromatin. Nuclear polylobation is characteristic and giant cells with very irregular nuclei may be present. In patients with early or smouldering chronic forms of the disease, the node may be only partially involved with infiltration of the paracortex by smaller cells and scattered giant cell forms resembling Hodgkin cells.

IMMUNOHISTOCHEMISTRY

Tumour cells express the T-cell antigens CD3 and CD5. They usually lack CD7 but stain strongly for the interleukin 2 (IL-2) receptor CD25. In most cases they are CD4+ and CD8− but exceptional cases are CD4− CD8+ or express both antigens. Large Hodgkin-like cells may express CD30, EBV-related antigens and even CD15, occasionally making the distinction from Hodgkin lymphoma difficult.

GENETICS

Apart from clonal rearrangement of the T-cell receptor genes, no specific genetic abnormality has been identified.

▲ BOX 6.12: Adult T-cell lymphoma/leukaemia: clinical features

- ▲ Confined to human T-cell leukaemia virus type I-positive individuals and concentrated in endemic areas
- ▲ Acute, chronic and smouldering clinical forms
- ▲ Leukaemia present in 60 per cent: diagnosis made on peripheral blood
- ▲ Hypercalcaemia in about 75 per cent
- ▲ Skin lesions common

● BOX 6.13: Adult T-cell lymphoma/leukaemia: morphology

- Cell size very variable but distinctive polylobation of nuclei
- Often shows retention of underlying reticulin structure of node
- May mimic other forms of T-cell lymphoma or Hodgkin lymphoma.

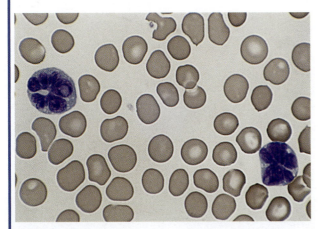

FIGURE 6.20 Adult T-cell leukaemia/lymphoma. Circulating neoplastic cells typically show complex lobation of the nuclei giving rise to the term 'flower cells'.

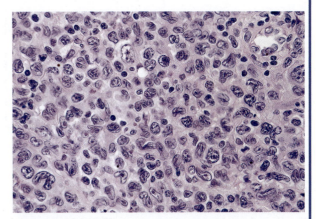

FIGURE 6.21 Adult T-cell leukaemia/lymphoma. In a typical case, the infiltrate is pleomorphic and many cells show nuclear folding and lobation.

DIFFERENTIAL DIAGNOSIS

Without immunohistochemistry, particularly in those tumours with a uniform cell type, the initial impression may be of a diffuse B-cell lymphoma. Mantle cell lymphoma may be favoured, if the cells are small or intermediate, or diffuse large B-cell lymphoma, if they are larger with more prominent nucleoli.

In those unusual cases with CD30+ Hodgkin-like cells, the distinction can be made by the co-expression of T-cell antigens.

The distinction between ATLL and other types of unspecified peripheral T-cell lymphoma may be very difficult unless the diagnosis of ATLL is considered. In non-endemic areas, it is an unlikely diagnosis and immunohistochemistry is not sufficiently specific to suggest it as a possibility. The distinctive nuclear polylobation is usually present and should provide the clue to the diagnosis.

Precursor T-lymphoblastic leukaemia/lymphoma is a consideration, particularly in younger patients. In general, the cells in this condition are much more uniform. Although some may show nuclear irregularity and folding, polylobation is not a feature. The immunophenotype varies (see page 51) but terminal deoxynucleotidyl transferase (TdT) is a very specific diagnostic marker.

T-Cell prolymphocytic leukaemia is discussed below. This condition has similar clinical features and the circulating cells may have very irregular nuclei. The immunophenotype is not distinctive, apart from those cases which co-express CD4 and CD8, but the cells lack the strong CD25 expression seen in ATLL.

survive for about a year after diagnosis. Like ATLL, it is a systemic disease in which leukaemia is associated with hepatosplenomegaly and generalized lymphadenopathy. The lymphocyte count is usually high, over 100×10^6, and there is associated anaemia and thrombocytopenia. The bone marrow is diffusely infiltrated and about 20 per cent of patients have skin infiltrates.

The diagnosis is usually made on the peripheral blood. The cells may resemble small lymphocytes or may be larger and 'prolymphocytic' with more prominent nucleoli. The nuclear outline may be round or irregular. A characteristic feature is the presence of cytoplasmic protrusions or blebs, seen in blood or marrow films.

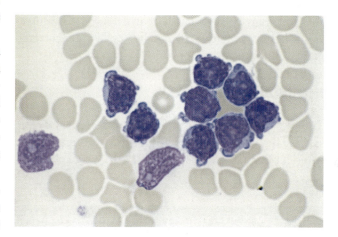

FIGURE 6.22 T-Cell prolymphocytic leukaemia. Leukaemic cells show nuclear irregularity and cytoplasmic blebs.

> ◆ **BOX 6.14: Adult T-cell lymphoma/leukaemia: immunohistochemistry**
>
> - CD3+ CD5+ CD7−
> - CD25++
> - Usually CD4+ CD8−
> - Occasionally CD30+

T-CELL PROLYMPHOCYTIC LEUKAEMIA

T-cell prolymphocytic leukaemia (T-PLL), previously known as T-cell chronic lymphocytic leukaemia, is a more aggressive disease than B-cell chronic lymphocytic leukaemia (Matutes et al. 1991). Although long survival is occasionally recorded, most patients only

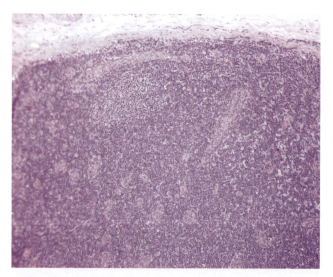

FIGURE 6.23 T-Cell prolymphocytic leukaemia. A low-power view of the node shows occasional spared follicles and high endothelial venules within the infiltrate.

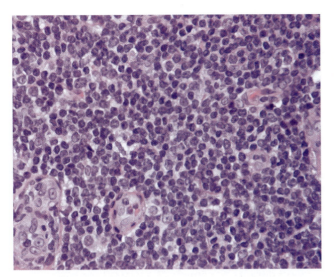

FIGURE 6.24 T-Cell prolymphocytic leukaemia. Cells are slightly larger than lymphocytes with slightly irregular nuclei and a single nucleolus.

HISTOLOGY

In lymph node biopsies, the appearances resemble B-cell small lymphocytic lymphoma but, in contrast to this disease, there are usually more residual follicles. Proliferation centres are absent and vessels, specifically high-endothelial venules, are more conspicuous. The cells are slightly larger than normal lymphocytes and have more open chromatin with small nucleoli. They show a variable degree of nuclear irregularity.

IMMUNOHISTOCHEMISTRY

The cells express the T-cell antigens CD3, CD5, and CD7. CD3 membrane staining may be weak but there is usually cytoplasmic staining. The majority of cases are CD4+, CD8−, a small number are CD8+, CD4− and some express both antigens.

GENETICS

In a majority of patients, there is an abnormality involving the TCRαβ locus at 14q11, usually with an inversion of chromosome 14, which causes juxtaposition of this locus with the TCL1 and TCL1b oncogenes. Abnormalities of chromosome 8 are also present in about 80 per cent of cases.

MYCOSIS FUNGOIDES/SÉZARY SYNDROME

Mycosis fungoides (MF) and Sézary syndrome (SS) are variants of cutaneous T-cell lymphoma in which there

is infiltration of the dermis and epidermis by neoplastic cells showing characteristic morphological features and epidermotropism. MF is usually an indolent disease, progressing over a period of years from erythematous patches resembling dermatitis or psoriasis, through a plaque phase to a tumour phase. SS is a rare, more aggressive variant in which there is generalized reddening of the skin (erythroderma), a leukaemic phase, with circulating atypical cells and bone marrow involvement, and lymphadenopathy. Involvement of extracutaneous organs is a late manifestation of MF and indicates advanced disease with a poor prognosis, and an average survival time of about 12 months from that point. In addition to the lymph nodes, the organs most often involved are the lungs, spleen and liver.

The characteristic cells in MF and SS are mature T-lymphocytes of helper cell type and are usually CD4 positive. Large and small variants are recognized. The small cells, sometimes known as Lutzner cells, are slightly larger than normal lymphocytes, and have deeply indented or convoluted nuclei, usually described as cerebriform. These are best seen in thin, plastic-embedded sections or by electron microscopy, but they can be appreciated in good-quality paraffin sections. Larger cells, or classical Sézary cells, have nuclei comparable in size to those of histiocytes. They are hyperchromatic and show even more marked nuclear irregularity and folding. Large and small cells are seen in both diseases, but small cells tend to predominate in the skin lesions of MF, at least in the early stages. In the late stages of the disease, blastic transformation may occur with the appearance of large CD30+ cells with less irregular nuclei and more prominent nucleoli. In SS, the circulating cells are usually of mixed small and large cell types.

LYMPH NODE HISTOLOGY

Assessment of lymph node involvement in MF is recognized to be a difficult and controversial area. It is important because it has been shown that lymph node involvement is associated with a worsening prognosis. Most patients with MF have some degree of lymphadenopathy, usually involving axillary and inguinal nodes draining the areas of involved skin. Histologically, the nodes show features of dermatopathic lymphadenopathy (see page 28) and it is against this background that involvement by neoplastic cells has to be assessed, as the two processes often co-exist. In nodes showing clear evidence of involvement, there is partial or complete infiltration by MF cells of both small and large cell type. The paracortical area is selectively involved initially, but then there is progression to total effacement with spread beyond the capsule and foci of

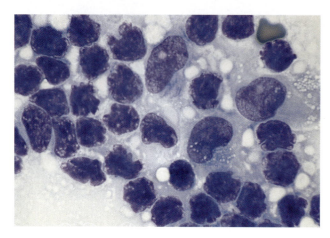

FIGURE 6.25 Mycosis fungoides/Sézary syndrome. In touch preparations, the cells show marked complex nuclear folding or convolutions.

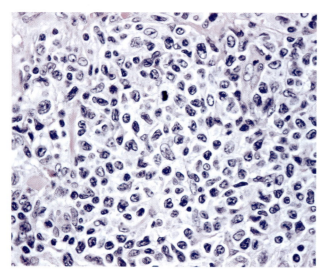

FIGURE 6.26 Mycosis fungoides/Sézary syndrome. In Grade 3 involvement, the infiltrating cells include large blasts and show considerable variation in size. Many have irregular folded nuclei.

> **BOX 6.15: Lymph node involvement in mycosis fungoides (MF) (Scheffer et al. 1980, Colby et al. 1981)**
>
> **GRADE 1: NO INVOLVEMENT BY MF**
> Dermatopathic lymphadenopathy. Scattered cerebriform lymphocytes but no clusters
>
> **GRADE 2: EARLY INVOLVEMENT BY MF**
> Focal obliteration of architecture with clusters of atypical cerebriform lymphocytes, often mainly paracortical in distribution
>
> **GRADE 3: MASSIVE INVOLVEMENT BY MF**
> Complete replacement of architecture with diffuse infiltrates of atypical cerebriform lymphocytes

IMMUNOHISTOCHEMISTRY

Neoplastic T-cells in MF and SS express CD3, CD5 and CD4. They are usually, but not invariably negative for CD8 and CD7. Large, CD30+ blasts may be present. Cytotoxic granule antigens, TIA-1 and granzyme, are usually negative but are sometimes expressed in more atypical cells in advanced lesions.

GENETICS

There is clonal rearrangement of T-cell receptor genes in most cases and this provides a useful way of assessing early nodal involvement. In those cases where there is doubt about lymph node involvement by microscopy, demonstration of T-cell clonality by PCR implies a worse prognosis.

ENTEROPATHY-TYPE T-CELL LYMPHOMA (ENTEROPATHY-ASSOCIATED T-CELL LYMPHOMA)

First described as malignant histiocytosis of the intestine, enteropathy-associated T-cell lymphoma (EATL) is now recognized as a form of T-cell lymphoma and is one of the more common forms seen in Europe. Its name derives from its close link to adult coeliac disease, which may be clinically occult prior to presentation of the lymphoma. A minority of patients show only minimal evidence of gluten enteropathy with an increase in intraepithelial lymphocytes. Patients, with or without a history of coeliac disease, usually present

necrosis. A confident diagnosis of early involvement is more difficult as small clusters of neoplastic T-cells may be difficult to recognize in a background of dermatopathic lymphadenopathy. The degree of atypia and nuclear irregularity may be insufficient to distinguish the neoplastic cells from benign T-cells and the immunophenotype is not specific. Good-quality thin sections from well-fixed material are essential in assessing the cell morphology. The WHO recommends a modified grading system for lymph node involvement in MF (Box 6.15).

Involved lymph nodes show similar features in SS. The assessment of early involvement may be less of a problem as there is usually diffuse infiltration by the tumour cells. Transformation to a large cell lymphoma may occur.

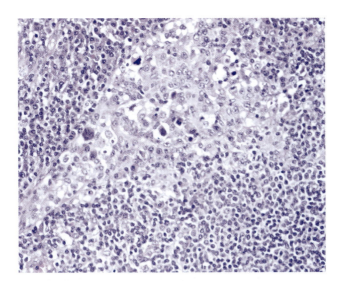

FIGURE 6.27 Enteropathy-associated T-cell lymphoma. In mesenteric nodes involved by EATL, the infiltrate is similar to that seen in the bowel wall. In this example of early involvement, the sinuses contain an infiltrate of pleomorphic cells.

with abdominal pain or small bowel perforation and are found to have ulceration of the small bowel, often with one or more tumour masses. Typically, the diagnosis is made on resected bowel but occasionally abdominal lymph nodes may be the only material available. The prognosis is very poor.

Neoplastic cells diffusely infiltrate the wall of the small bowel. Most frequently, these are intermediate to large with rounded or irregular nuclei and prominent nucleoli. The cell population may appear polymorphic owing to the presence of inflammatory cells, including eosinophils and histiocytes. Some tumours show more marked pleomorphism with multinucleate cells. The adjacent mucosa often shows the changes of coeliac disease and large numbers of intraepithelial lymphocytes are typically present. In a small subset of cases in which the features of coeliac disease are lacking, the tumour cells are smaller and more monotonous with more darkly staining nuclei (Wright 1997).

LYMPH NODE HISTOLOGY

Involved mesenteric lymph nodes are often completely effaced by a infiltrate similar to that seen in the bowel wall but the degree of infiltration is variable and, in nodes showing early involvement, the tumour cells may show a sinus pattern of spread.

IMMUNOHISTOCHEMISTRY

The tumour cells typically express CD3, CD7, and larger, more anaplastic cells express CD30 to a variable

degree (Wright 1997). CD5 and CD4 are negative and CD8 is usually negative except in the small group of tumours consisting of small to intermediate-sized cells, which express CD8 and CD56 (Chott *et al.* 1998). The cytotoxic granule markers, TIA-1, granzyme and perforin, are positive.

DIFFERENTIAL DIAGNOSIS

In the unusual event of there being no definite evidence of small bowel pathology, or if only a needle core biopsy is available, EATL has to be distinguished from other forms of T-cell lymphoma. Depending on the morphological features, these include ALCL and PTLU. ALCL is a consideration if the tumour shows considerable pleomorphism. The immunophenotype is similar, with the important exception of CD3 and CD7, which are usually negative in ALCL. In those tumours showing more uniform cell morphology with weak or absent CD30 expression, the distinction from PTLU is difficult but the presence of cytotoxic granule-associated proteins points to EATL.

BLASTIC NK-CELL LYMPHOMA

Blastic NK-cell lymphoma is rare. It is a tumour of older people and usually presents as cutaneous nodules. Lymph nodes, spleen and bone marrow are often involved, and the disease may be disseminated at presentation with circulating malignant cells and pancytopaenia. There is some evidence that it may be a heterogeneous disease with cutaneous and non-cutaneous subtypes (Suzuki *et al.* 2005). The prognosis is poor despite an initially good response to chemotherapy and relapse is often in the central nervous system.

HISTOLOGY

Lesions in the skin and elsewhere are characterized by an infiltrate of fairly uniform medium-sized cells. In a minority of cases, the cell population is more mixed with larger forms. They resemble lymphoblastic lymphoma or acute myeloid leukaemia, even to the extent that a single-file or 'Indian-file' pattern of infiltration may be seen. The chromatin pattern is described as lacey or dispersed, and nucleoli are inconspicuous.

Although described as blastic NK-cell lymphoma in the WHO classification, the cell of origin is uncertain. There is some evidence that it derives from the dendritic, type 2 plasmacytoid monocyte.

IMMUNOHISTOCHEMISTRY

Tumour cells are typically positive for CD4 and CD56, and this gives rise to one of the alternative terms, 'agranular CD4+, CD56+ haematodermic neoplasm' (Petrella *et al.* 2002). The usual lymphoid and myeloid markers (including CD3 and CD5) are lacking and the typical immunophenotype is: CD45 weakly positive, CD45RA positive and CD123 (IL-Rα) positive. CD38, CD68 and CD7 are usually positive.

DIFFERENTIAL DIAGNOSIS

The diagnosis of blastic NK-cell lymphoma should be considered if the immunophenotype is typical and lymphoblastic lymphoma or myeloid leukaemia can be excluded. PCR can be used to confirm that there is no TCR gene rearrangement.

REFERENCES

Adam P, Katzenberger T, Seeberger H, *et al.* 2003 A case of large B-cell lymphoma of plasmablastic type associated with the t(2;5)(p23;q35) chromosomal translocation. *American Journal of Surgical Pathology* 27: 1473–1476.

Anon. 1997 A clinical evaluation of the International Lymphoma Study Group classification of Non-Hodgkin's lymphoma. The Non-Hodgkin's Lymphoma Classification Project. *Blood* 89: 3908–3918.

Ascani S, Zinzani PL, Gherlinzoni F, *et al.* 1997 Peripheral T-cell lymphomas. Clinico-pathologic study of 168 cases diagnosed according to the REAL Classification. *Annals of Oncology* 8: 583–592.

Attygale AD, Diss TC, Munson P, *et al.* 2004 CD10 expression in extranodal dissemination of angioimmunoblastic T-cell lymphoma. *American Journal of Surgical Pathology* 28: 54–61.

Attygale AD, Jehani R, Diss TC, *et al.* 2002 Neoplastic T-cells in angioimmunoblastic T-cell lymphoma express CD10. *Blood* 99: 627–633.

Benharroch D, Meguerian-Bedoyan Z, Lamant L, *et al.* 1998 ALK-positive lymphoma a single disease with a broad spectrum of morphology. *Blood* 91: 2076–2084.

Bonzheim I, Geissinger E, Roth S, *et al.* 2004 Anaplastic large cell lymphomas lack the expression of T-cell receptor molecules or molecules of proximal T-cell receptor signalling. *Blood* 104: 3358–3360.

Cheuk W, Hill RW, Bacchi C, Dias MA, Chan JK 2000 Hypocellular anaplastic large cell lymphoma mimicking inflammatory lesions of lymph nodes. *American Journal of Surgical Pathology* 24: 1537–1543.

Chott A, Haedicke W, Mosberger I, *et al.* 1998 Most CD56+ intestinal lymphomas are CD8+ CD5− T-cell lymphomas of monomorphic small to medium size histology. *American Journal of Pathology* 153: 1483–1490.

Colby TV, Burke JS, Hoppe RT 1981 Lymph node biopsy in mycosis fungoides. *Cancer* 47: 351–359.

Delsol G, Lamont L, Mariame B, *et al.* 1997 A new subtype of large B-cell lymphoma expressing the ALK kinase and lacking the 2;5 translocation. *Blood* 89: 1483–1490.

Dogan A 2003 Angioimmunoblastic T-cell lymphoma. *British Journal of Haematology* 121: 681–691.

Geissinger E, Odenwald T, Lee SS, *et al.* 2004 Nodal peripheral T-cell lymphomas and, in particular, their lymphoepithelioid (Lennert's) variant are often derived from CD8(+) cytotoxic T-cells. *Virchows Archiv* 445: 334–343.

Harris NL, Jaffe ES, Stein H, *et al.* 1994 A revised European–American classification of lymphoid neoplasms: a proposal from the International Lymphoma Study Group. *Blood* 84: 1361–1392.

Jaffe ES 2001 Anaplastic large cell lymphoma: the shifting sands of diagnostic haematopathology. *Modern Pathology* 14: 219–228.

Jaffe ES, Harris NL, Stein H, Vardiman JW (eds) 2001 *Tumours of the Haematopoietic and Lymphoid Tissues.* Lyon: IARC Press.

Jones D, Jorgensen JL, Shahsafaei A, *et al.* 1998 Characteristic proliferations of reticular and dendritic cells in angioimmunoblastic lymphoma. *American Journal of Surgical Pathology* 22: 956–964.

Matutes E, Brito-Babapulle V, Swansbury J, *et al.* 1991 Clinical and laboratory features of 78 cases of T-prolymphocytic leukaemia. *Blood* 78: 3269–3274.

Morris SW 2003 ALK in NHL: to B (cell) or not to B (cell)? Characterization of the entity 'ALK+ DLBCL' (editorial). *Blood* 102: 2316–2317.

Onciu M, Behm FG, Raimondi SC, *et al.* 2003 ALK-positive anaplastic large cell lymphoma with leukaemic peripheral blood involvement is a clinicopathological entity with an unfavourable prognosis. Report of three cases and review of the literature. *American Journal of Clinical Pathology* 120: 617–625.

Ottaviani G, Buesco-Ramos CE, Seilstad K, *et al.* 2004 The role of the perifollicular sinus in determining the complex immunoarchitecture of angioimmunoblastic T-cell lymphoma. *American Journal of Surgical Pathology* 28: 1632–1640.

Petrella T, Comeau MR, Maynadie M, et al. 2002 Agranular CD4+ CD56+ haematodermic neoplasm (blastic NK-cell lymphoma) originates from a population of CD56+ precursor cells related to plasmacytoid monocytes. American Journal of Surgical Pathology **26:** 852–862.

Quintanilla-Martinez L, Fend F, Rodriquez-Martinez L, et al. 1999 Peripheral T-cell lymphoma with Reed–Sternberg-like cells of B-cell phenotype and genotype associated with Epstein–Barr virus infection. American Journal of Surgical Pathology **23:** 1233–1240.

Ree HJ, Kadin ME, Kikuchi M, et al. 1998 Angioimmunoblastic lymphoma (AILD-type T-cell lymphoma) with hyperplastic germinal centers. American Journal of Surgical Pathology **22:** 643–655.

Rudiger T, Ichinohasama R, Ott MM, et al. 2000 Peripheral T-cell lymphoma with distinct perifollicular growth pattern. A distinct subtype of T-cell lymphoma? American Journal of Surgical Pathology **24:** 117–122.

Scheffer E, Meijer CJ, vanVloten WA 1980 Dermatopathic lymphadenopathy and lymph node involvement in mycosis fungoides. Cancer **45:** 137–148.

Shimoyama M 1991 Diagnostic criteria and classification of clinical subtypes of adult T-cell leukaemia-lymphoma. A report from the Lymphoma Study Group (1984–87). British Journal of Haematology **79:** 428–437.

Stein H, Mason DY, Gerdes J, et al. 1985 The expression of the Hodgkin disease associated antigen Ki-1 in reactive and neoplastic lymphoid tissue: evidence that Reed–Sternberg cells and histiocytic malignancies are derived from activated lymphoid cells. Blood **66:** 848–858.

Stein H, Foss H-D, Durkop H, et al. 2000 CD30+ anaplastic large cell lymphoma: a review of its histopathologic, genetic, and clinical features. Blood **96:** 3681–3695.

Suchi T, Lennert K, Tu LY, et al. 1987 Histopathology and immunohistochemistry of peripheral T-cell lymphomas: a proposal for their classification. Journal of Clinical Pathology **40:** 995–1015.

Suzuki R, Nakamura S, Suzumiya J et al. 2005 Blastic natural killer cell lymphoma/leukemia (CD56-positive blastic tumor). Cancer **104:** 1022–1031.

Wright DH 1997 Enteropathy-associated T-cell lymphoma. Cancer Surveys **30:** 249–261.

IMMUNODEFICIENCY-ASSOCIATED LYMPHO-PROLIFERATIVE DISORDERS

LYMPHOMATOID GRANULOMATOSIS

Lymphomatoid granulomatosis is included in the World Health Organization (WHO) Classification as a mature B-cell proliferation of uncertain malignant potential. It is an uncommon disease that almost invariably involves the lungs, frequently involves other extranodal sites (skin, brain, kidney, liver) but rarely involves lymph nodes. The infiltrate is composed of small T-cells and variable numbers of Epstein–Barr (EBV)-positive B-cells, sometimes showing polymorphism. An angiocentric and angiodestructive growth pattern is frequently seen and this may result in areas of infarction. Vascular damage may also be induced by EBV-mediated chemokine release.

Lymphomatoid granulomatosis is graded as follows.

- *Grade I:* less than 5 EBV-positive large B-cells per high-power field; rarely shows necrosis.
- *Grade II:* 5–20 EBV-positive large B-cells per high power field; necrosis more commonly seen.
- *Grade III:* large numbers of EBV-positive B-cells forming confluent sheets in some areas; variable numbers of small T-cells; necrosis common.

(The B-cells of Grade II and Grade III disease are usually clonal.) This subtype should be regarded as a variant of diffuse large B-cell lymphoma.

Patients with lymphomatoid granulomatosis usually show an underlying inherited or acquired immunodeficiency state. Those that do not have a specific immunodeficiency disorder usually show evidence of impaired immune function. The disease course may fluctuate spontaneously or in response to immunomodulation.

DIFFERENTIAL DIAGNOSIS

Lymphomatoid granulomatosis differs from post-transplant lymphoproliferative disorder, polymorphic, in its clinical (predominantly pulmonary) manifestation. Histologically, post-transplant lymphoproliferative disorder, polymorphic shows a range of B-cells from plasma cells to immunoblasts, whereas lymphomatoid granulomatosis has a predominant background of small T-cells.

The B-cells in T-cell/histiocyte-rich B-cell lymphoma may be EBV positive, but this lymphoma usually presents as nodal disease, and does not show the angio-invasive and angiodestructive features of lymphomatoid granulomatosis.

LYMPHOPROLIFERATIVE DISEASES ASSOCIATED WITH PRIMARY IMMUNODEFICIENCY DISEASES

The primary immune disorders are rare and have diverse underlying pathologies. They occur predominantly in childhood, although common variable immunodeficiency is seen in adults. Primary immune disorders are associated with polymorphic, polyclonal lymphoproliferations, including lymphomatous granulomatosis, and leukaemias and lymphomas. The underlying pathogenesis of these lymphoproliferations in most cases appears to be impaired T-cell immunity to EBV leading to B-cell proliferation and eventually to neoplasia. Most neoplasms occur at extranodal sites.

Fatal infectious mononucleosis is seen in patients with X-linked lymphoproliferation (Duncan syndrome) and with severe combined immunodeficiency (SCID). Infection with EBV is associated with unrestrained proliferation of EBV-positive plasmacytoid and immunoblastic cells at nodal and extranodal sites. Death may be due to haemophagocytic syndrome, pancytopaenia and infection.

Diffuse large B-cell lymphoma and Burkitt lymphoma are the most common lymphomas complicating primary immunodeficiency diseases.

T-cell leukaemia/lymphoma occurs more commonly in ataxia telangiectasia (abnormal DNA repair mechanism) than B-cell lymphoma.

Hodgkin lymphoma has rarely been reported in patients with primary immunodeficiency.

LYMPHOMAS ASSOCIATED WITH INFECTION BY THE HUMAN IMMUNODEFICIENCY VIRUS

Patients with human immunodeficiency virus (HIV) infection have an increased incidence of malignant lymphomas; although this incidence may be falling with the introduction of effective antiretroviral therapy. Malignant lymphomas constitute an acquired immune deficiency syndrome (AIDS)-defining feature in HIV-positive patients.

Two rare lymphomas, primary effusion lymphoma and plasmablastic lymphoma of the oral cavity, are specifically associated with AIDS. These tumours are not associated with lymphadenopathy.

The commonest lymphomas seen in AIDS patients are diffuse large B-cell lymphoma (DLBCL) and Burkitt lymphoma (BL). These most frequently present with extranodal tumours, most commonly in the gastrointestinal tract. The WHO classification recognizes a variant of Burkitt lymphoma 'with plasmacytoid differentiation', which is reported to be more common in AIDS patients. It is debatable whether such tumours should be categorized as BL and, if they are, whether they would be better consigned to the category of 'atypical BL'.

There is an increased incidence of Hodgkin lymphoma in patients with HIV infection, with a greater prevalence of the poor prognosis subtypes (mixed cellularity and lymphocyte depleted) than is seen in immunocompetent patients.

POST-TRANSPLANT LYMPHOPROLIFERATIVE DISORDERS

The incidence of post-transplant lymphoproliferative disorders (PTLD) varies with the type of allograft and the immunosuppressive regime used. Historically, renal transplants have a risk of less than 1 per cent, whereas, following cardiac transplantation, the risk is 7 per cent. The risk of PTLD following bone marrow transplantation is less than 1 per cent except in patients with HLA mismatch with high levels of immunosuppression. PTLD is of host origin in 90 per cent of cases and donor origin in 10 per cent, except following bone marrow transplantation when almost all cases are of donor origin.

As with other immunodeficiency-associated lymphoproliferations, impaired T-cell immunity to EBV appears to be a major causal factor in PTLD. Patients who acquire EBV infection following transplantation are at greater risk of developing PTLD than those who already have immunity to the virus. Approximately 20 per cent of PTLD are EBV negative. These occur later (4–5 years post-transplant) than EBV-positive cases (6–10 months post-transplant). Both may regress following reduction in immunosuppression. PTLD may be nodal or extranodal including involvement of the allograft itself.

PLASMACYTIC HYPERPLASIA AND INFECTIOUS MONONUCLEOSIS-LIKE PTLD

These proliferations typically involve lymph nodes and the tissues of Waldeyer's ring. They occur most commonly among young patients who were EBV negative at the time of transplantation.

Histology usually shows partial preservation of the normal nodal structure with a proliferation of plasma cells or of blast cells, as seen in primary immunodeficiency-associated fatal infectious mononucleosis.

POLYMORPHIC PTLD

These proliferations usually show loss of the normal nodal architecture with a mixed infiltrate of small lymphocytes with angulated nuclei, plasma cells and immunoblasts. Bizarre cells may be seen and there may be areas of necrosis. Such cases may regress following reduction of immunosuppression or may require treatment for lymphoma. Immunoglobulin gene analysis will usually show the proliferation to be clonal.

MONOMORPHIC PTLD

These proliferations resemble lymphomas and should be reported as such, although PTLD should appear in the diagnosis since they may regress following reduction of immunosuppression. The majority of cases are of large B-cell lymphomas; less commonly Burkitt lymphoma.

T-cell PTLD is much less common than B-cell PTLD. It is often an extranodal lymphoma, such as subcutaneous panniculitis-like T-cell lymphoma or hepatosplenic T-cell lymphoma. Post-transplant Hodgkin lymphoma has been reported. This should not be confused with other PTLD containing occasional CD30-positive multinucleated cells.

METHOTREXATE-ASSOCIATED LYMPHOPROLIFERATIVE DISORDERS

A relatively small number of patients receiving long-term methotrexate therapy for autoimmune disease (rheumatoid arthritis, psoriasis, dermatomyositis) have been reported to develop malignant lymphomas or lymphoma-like proliferations. The commonest of these is diffuse large B-cell lymphoma, but almost a third of cases have Hodgkin lymphoma or Hodgkin-like lesions (Kamel *et al.* 1996, Jaffe *et al.* 2001). The increased incidence of malignant lymphomas in patients with autoimmune diseases must be taken into account when interpreting these findings. However, the response of many of the reported cases to the withdrawal of methotrexate therapy suggests that the immunosuppressive drug does have a role in lymphoma development in some cases.

REFERENCES

Jaffe ES, Harris NL, Stein H, Vardiman JW 2001 Methotrexate-associated lymphoproliferative disorders. In: *Pathology and Genetics of Tumours of Haematopoietic and Lymphoid Tissues*. Lyon: IARC Press, pp. 270–271.

Kamel OW, Weiss LM, van de Rijn M, *et al.* 1996 Hodgkin's disease and lymphoproliferations resembling Hodgkin's disease in patients receiving long-term methotrexate therapy. *American Journal of Surgical Pathology* **20**: 1279–1287.

8 HODGKIN LYMPHOMA

INTRODUCTION

Hodgkin lymphoma (HL) occupies an enigmatic place among malignant lymphomas. Thomas Hodgkin was appointed to the post of Inspector of the Dead and Curator of the Museum at Guy's Hospital in 1826. In his role as a morbid anatomist, he noted a peculiar appearance of the lymph nodes and spleen in six patients, and was shown paintings of a similar case from France by his friend Robert Carswell, the first professor of pathology at University College Hospital. Hodgkin presented details of these cases in two lectures given to the Medical-Chirurgical Society in 1832 that were subsequently published in the transactions of that society under the title 'On some morbid appearances of the absorbent glands and spleen'. This paper would have probably faded into obscurity had not Sir Samuel Wilks, a distinguished physician at Guy's Hospital, described similar cases between 1856 and 1877 and, noting Dr Hodgkin's precedence, named them as Hodgkin's disease.

In 1926, an American pathologist, Herbert Fox, traced tissue from three of the six cases described by Hodgkin. Histology of these tissues showed two to be what he considered to be Hodgkin's disease and one to be a non-Hodgkin lymphoma (NHL). It is amazing that, from such modest beginnings, all malignant lymphomas are categorized as either HL or NHL at the beginning of the twenty-first century.

In the twentieth century, the Reed–Sternberg (RS) cell was recognized as the hallmark cell of Hodgkin's disease. Following a spate of reports of RS cells in a diverse range of reactive and neoplastic conditions, it became accepted that the RS cell was diagnostic of Hodgkin's disease only if it was in a background of reactive cells characteristic of one of the subtypes of this disease. Immunohistochemistry further refined the diagnosis of Hodgkin's disease with the identification of antigens characteristic of RS cells. There remain, however, grey areas in which the distinction between HL and NHL is difficult. The feature that distinguishes most cases of HL from NHL is that the neoplastic cells (Hodgkin and RS cells) usually form a minority population within the tumour, sometimes accounting for less than 1 per cent of the cells. The reactive cells (lymphocytes, plasma cells, histiocytes, neutrophils, eosinophils, fibroblasts) appear to be attracted into the proliferation by cytokines and chemokines secreted by or induced by the neoplastic cells (Teruya-Feldstein *et al.* 1999).

The nature of the RS cell remained a mystery for most of the twentieth century with many candidates being proposed as the cell of origin. Immunohistochemistry and molecular genetics indicate that the majority of RS cells are derived from germinal centre B-cells that have lost their ability to synthesize immunoglobulin and to express many B-cell antigens. It remains a possibility that a minority of cases of HL have RS cells of different origins.

BOX 8.1: WHO classification of Hodgkin lymphoma

Nodular lymphocyte-predominant Hodgkin lymphoma
Classical Hodgkin lymphoma
- Nodular sclerosis classical Hodgkin lymphoma
- Lymphocyte-rich classical Hodgkin lymphoma
- Mixed cellularity classical Hodgkin lymphoma
- Lymphocyte-depleted classical Hodgkin lymphoma

Hodgkin lymphoma accounts for approximately 10 per cent of all lymphomas. It shows a bimodal age distribution with the majority of cases occurring in young adult life. Cervical lymph nodes are the commonest site of presentation and of biopsy. Other axial lymph node groups may be involved but involvement of the mesenteric nodes is rare. The spleen is involved in approximately 20 per cent of cases but other extra-nodal tumour is uncommon except in advanced stage disease. The mode of spread of HL, by contiguity, is a feature that differentiates it from most NHLs, which tend to be more widely disseminated. This contiguous mode of spread provides the rationale for the Ann Arbor staging system on which the treatment of HL is based.

Within the World Health Organization (WHO) classification of HL there are two entities, nodular lymphocyte-predominant Hodgkin lymphoma (NLPHL) and classical Hodgkin lymphoma, which differ from each other with respect to their clinical features, immunohistochemistry and molecular genetics. There is an argument for placing NLPHL amongst the B-cell non-Hodgkin lymphomas. However, the WHO Working group felt that, at the present time, NLPHL should remain as a subtype of HL pending further investigation (Box 8.1).

NODULAR LYMPHOCYTE-PREDOMINANT HODGKIN LYMPHOMA

Nodular lymphocyte-predominant Hodgkin lymphoma is an uncommon neoplasm accounting for less than 5 per cent of all cases of HL. It was almost certainly not represented among the cases described by Thomas Hodgkin, and it differs from classic HL in its clinical behaviour, histology, immunohistochemistry and molecular genetics. Nevertheless, it has in the past been confused with classical HL, particularly with lymphocyte-rich classical HL, and, at least for the time being, it has been categorized as HL in the WHO classification.

Nodular lymphocyte-predominant Hodgkin lymphoma shows a marked male predominance. It can occur from childhood to late adult life but shows a peak incidence in the fourth decade of life. The majority of patients present with lymphadenopathy in the cervical, axillary or, less commonly, inguinal regions. Involvement of other sites is uncommon. Lymphadenopathy may be of long duration. Over 80 per cent of patients have Stage I or II disease and, in some patients, the excision biopsy alone may be curative. In most patients, the disease runs an indolent course in which recurrence is common but disease-related death is rare. Five per cent or more patients have advanced disease, which is more often progressive and fatal. The number of such cases and their nature needs re-evaluation in view of the frequent misdiagnosis of lymphocyte-rich classical HL and T-cell/histiocyte-rich B-cell lymphoma as NLPHL, and the continuing confusion between these entities (Anagnostopoulos et al. 2000).

Rarely, NLPHL may show synchronous or metachronous association with progressive transformation of germinal centres (PTGC). The majority of cases of PTGC, however, run an entirely benign course, although recurrence is not uncommon. A small percentage of cases of NLPHL (3–5 per cent) have been reported to progress to diffuse large B-cell lymphoma and rare patients in whom NLPHD occurs subsequent to a diffuse large B-cell lymphoma have been recorded. The diffuse large B-cell lymphomas associated with NLPHL have been reported to run a more favourable course than primary diffuse large B-cell lymphoma.

Classical cases of NLPHL have a nodular growth pattern with large, relatively uniform nodules displacing the normal nodal structures, which may be seen as a compressed rim at one end of the biopsy. The nodularity may be highlighted by a reticulin stain or by immunohistochemistry for B-cells or dendritic reticulum cells. Some cases of NLPHL show a partial diffuse growth pattern and it is debateable whether NLPHL can have an entirely diffuse growth pattern. The presence of diffuse T-cell-rich areas has been found to be more common in patients with recurrent disease. The current WHO classification of lymphomas demands that at least one nodule is recognized for the diagnosis of NLPHL.

The tumour cells of NLPHL are frequently referred to as L&H cells after the Lukes and Butler classification, which used the designation lymphocytic and/or histiocytic (L&H) predominance Hodgkin's disease for what is now known as NLPHL. L&H cells are usually found within the nodules but may be internodular. They may be scanty or abundant. The nuclei are open with fine chromatin and are typically multilobated (popcorn cells). Nucleoli are clearly visible but are rarely as large as those seen in classic RS cells. For many years, it was the rule that classic RS cells should be seen before a diagnosis of NLPHL was made. It is now recognized that classic RS cells do not occur in NLPHL.

The background cells are composed predominantly of small lymphocytes. Histiocytes, singly or in clusters, may be seen, but plasma cells are uncommon and neutrophils and eosinophils are not a feature of NLPHL. Varying degrees of banded sclerosis may be present and, rarely, residual follicle centres are recognizable.

IMMUNOPHENOTYPE

The neoplastic cells of NLPHL are B-cells. They express CD45, CD20, CD79a and BCL-6. They are positive for the B-cell transcription factors BSAP, BOB-1 and Oct-2, and, in well-fixed tissues, J chain as well as immunoglobulin heavy and light chains can be detected.

Staining for CD15 is almost invariably negative and staining for CD30 is usually negative or weak. Careful evaluation will usually show that any CD30-positive cells are background mononuclear cells similar to those seen around reactive follicles. Most L&H cells show strong nuclear staining for Ki67 indicating that they are in cycle. Approximately 50 per cent express epithelial membrane antigen (EMA). L&H cells do not contain EBERs, neither do they express EBV-associated antigens.

The background cells are predominantly polyclonal small B-lymphocytes. However, within the sea of small B-cells, the L&H cells are surrounded in a rosette by small T-cells. The number of small T-cells appear to increase as the disease progresses and they are often the predominant population within the diffuse areas. A variable proportion of the T-cells, including those in a rosette around the L&H cells, express CD57. Each nodule is filled with an expanded network of follicular dendritic cells, identifiable with CD21 and CD23. Staining for this network and for B-cells may identify an underlying nodular growth pattern in what may appear to be a diffuse proliferation on routine histology.

GENETICS

Analysis of the immunogenetics of L&H cells has only been possible since the introduction of micromanipulation to isolate single cells. The L&H cells in any one case show monoclonal rearrangements of the immunoglobulin genes. The variable region genes show a high degree of mutation and show ongoing mutations characteristic of follicle centre B-cells. The immunoglobulin rearrangements appear to be functional.

DIFFERENTIAL DIAGNOSIS

The nodular form of NLPHL is a distinctive proliferation. PTGC is the only entity likely to come into the differential diagnosis. In PTGC, germinal centres are infiltrated and expanded by small B-mantle cells and may resemble the individual nodules of NLPHL. Also, small clusters or individual centroblasts are surrounded by small lymphocytes, but popcorn cells are not seen. The formation of a rosette around popcorn cells by T-lymphocytes, a feature of NLPHL, is rarely seen in progressive transformation of germinal centres (Nguyen et al. 1999). These two conditions are usually easily distinguished on low-power microscopy, since PTGC involves one or more follicles within a reactive lymph node, whereas NLPHL displaces and compresses the residual nodal tissue.

The differentiation of NLPHL from classical HL is important from a patient management point of view and can be difficult. In well-fixed tissue, L&H cells can usually be differentiated from classic RS cells or lacunar cells on the basis of their morphology. They can also be differentiated on the basis of their immunohistochemistry.

▲ BOX 8.2: Nodular lymphocyte-predominant Hodgkin lymphoma: clinical features

- ▲ Peak age incidence in fourth decade of life
- ▲ Male predominance
- ▲ Most common presentation with enlarged cervical, axillary or, less commonly, inguinal lymph nodes
- ▲ Lymphadenopathy may be of long duration
- ▲ Most patients have Stage I or Stage II disease
- ▲ Recurrence common but rarely fatal
- ▲ Three to five per cent develop diffuse large B-cell lymphoma

The differentiation between NLPHL with a predominantly diffuse growth pattern from T-cell/histiocyte rich B-cell lymphoma (T/HRBCL) is particularly difficult. It has been suggested that T/HRBCL may be an aggressive variant of NLPHL, although comparative genomic hybridization studies of cells obtained by microdissection suggests that these are separate entities (Franke *et al.* 2002). The finding of one or more areas of nodular growth will favour a diagnosis of NLPHL. However, if the tissue selected for histology does not include that nodule, or if the progression to a diffuse growth pattern is total, this means of differentiation will not be available. One study has shown that a background population of T-lymphocytes rich in cytotoxic (TIA-1-positive) cells favours a diagnosis of T/HRBCL or classic HL, whereas increased numbers of CD57 cells together with expanded networks of follicular dendritic cells support a diagnosis of NLPHL (Boudova *et al.* 2003).

● **BOX 8.3: Nodular lymphocyte-predominant Hodgkin lymphoma: morphology**

- Nodular or nodular and diffuse growth pattern
- Neoplastic cells (L&H cells) often have multi-lobated nuclei (popcorn cells)
- L&H cells may be scanty or abundant
- Background cells mainly small lymphocytes and histiocytes

- Histiocytes may have epithelioid morphology and form clusters or ring nodules
- Neutrophils and eosinophils absent
- Plasma cells usually scanty
- Sclerosis may be present

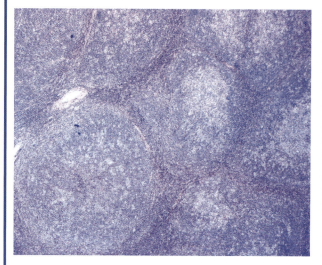

FIGURE 8.1 Nodular lymphocyte-predominant Hodgkin lymphoma. Low-power view, showing nodular growth pattern.

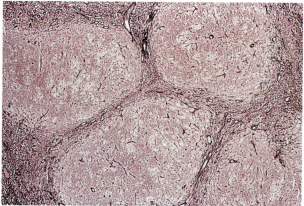

FIGURE 8.2 Section of nodular lymphocyte-predominant Hodgkin lymphoma, stained for reticulin, showing the characteristic nodular growth pattern.

◆ **BOX 8.4: Nodular lymphocyte-predominant Hodgkin lymphoma: immunohistochemistry**

L&H CELLS

- ◆ CD45 positive
- ◆ CD20 and CD79a positive
- ◆ B-cell transcription factors – BOB-1, Oct-2 and BSAP positive
- ◆ J-chain positive; immunoglobulin heavy and light chains may be detected
- ◆ EMA positive in 50 per cent of cases
- ◆ CD15 negative, CD30 weak or negative

BACKGROUND CELLS

- ◆ Predominantly polyclonal small B-cells
- ◆ Small T-cells rosette L&H cells and form more of the background cells in diffuse areas
- ◆ Many of the T-cells express CD57
- ◆ CD21 identifies expanded dendritic cell network within nodules

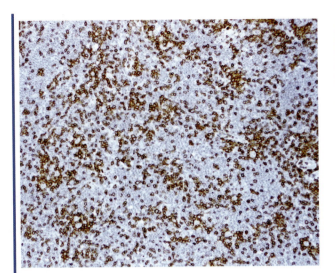

FIGURE 8.3 Nodular lymphocyte-predominant Hodgkin lymphoma, showing the centre of a nodule stained for CD3. Note the T-cell rosetting of the popcorn cells.

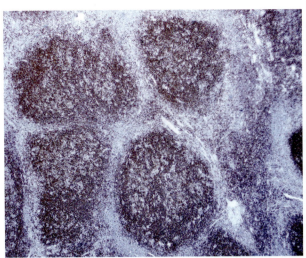

FIGURE 8.4 Nodular lymphocyte-predominant Hodgkin lymphoma, stained for CD20, showing nodular proliferation composed predominantly of B-cells.

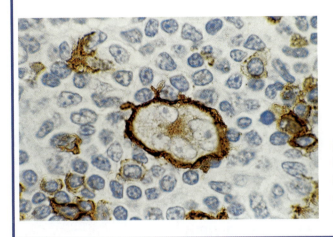

FIGURE 8.5 Section of nodular lymphocyte-predominant Hodgkin lymphoma, stained for CD20, showing a strongly labelled multinucleated 'popcorn cell' surrounded by unstained T-lymphocytes. Cytoplasmic spikes from the 'popcorn cell' extend between the T-cells.

CLASSICAL HODGKIN LYMPHOMA

Histologically, classical Hodgkin lymphoma (CHL) is composed of variable proportions of RS cells, mononuclear Hodgkin cells and their variants (H/RS cells) set in a background population of small lymphocytes (predominantly T-cells), eosinophils, neutrophils, histiocytes, plasma cells, fibroblasts and collagen. The four subtypes of CHL, largely defined by this background population, show broad differences in their clinical characteristics and such features as EBV association. The immunophenotype and molecular genetics of the H/RS cells are identical in all the subtypes of CHL.

Classical Hodgkin lymphoma may occur at all ages from early childhood onwards. It shows a bimodal age distribution with a peak incidence between 15 and 35 years, and a later less well-defined peak in older age.

There is an increased incidence of CHL in patients with a previous history of infectious mononucleosis and in patients with human immunodeficiency virus (HIV) infection.

Classical Hodgkin lymphoma typically involves the axial lymph node groups (cervical, mediastinal, axillary, inguinal and para-aortic) and occurs rarely in the mesenteric lymph nodes. Mediastinal tumour, which may involve lymph nodes or thymus, occurs in 60 per cent of patients with nodular sclerosing Hodgkin lymphoma (NSHL). Splenic tumour is found in 20 per cent of patients, and appears to be necessary for further haematogenous spread to the liver and bone marrow. Primary involvement of Waldeyer's ring (tonsils and adenoids) and the gastrointestinal tract is rare.

Classical Hodgkin lymphoma is staged, according to its spread, broadly as follows.

- *Stage I*: involvement of a single lymph node group or lymphoid structure.
- *Stage II*: involvement of two or more lymph node groups, or lymphoid structures, on the same side of the diaphragm.
- *Stage III*: involvement of lymph node groups, or lymphoid structures, on both sides of the diaphragm.
- *Stage IV*: involvement of extranodal sites, such as liver and bone marrow.

Patients with CHL may experience a number of systemic symptoms. Fever, drenching night sweats and weight loss are categorized as 'B-symptoms' and have adverse prognostic significance.

The classic RS cell is binucleate or has a bilobed nucleus. Each nucleus or nuclear lobe contains a large eosinophilic nucleolus giving the cell an 'owl-eye' appearance. Delicate strands of chromatin often radiate from the nucleolus to the well-defined nuclear membrane. In Giemsa-stained preparations, the cytoplasm is basophilic. Mononuclear Hodgkin cells have similar nuclear and cytoplasmic features and some of them probably represent RS cells cut in a plane that shows only one nucleus or nuclear lobe. Shrunken, pyknotic H/RS cells are frequently encountered in CHL; they are referred to as mummified cells. Variant forms of H/RS cells, known as lacunar cells, are found in NSHL and are described in the section on that subtype.

IMMUNOHISTOCHEMISTRY

In almost all cases of HL, at least a proportion of the H/RS cells express CD30. This takes the form of membrane staining with additional positivity in the Golgi region. CD15 shows a similar staining pattern in 75–85 per cent of cases. In the region of 10 per cent of cases of HL, the H/RS cells show variable CD20 expression. CD79a is less frequently expressed. H/RS cells are CD45 negative, although this is often difficult to determine because of the close apposition of CD45-positive lymphocytes forming a rosette. H/RS cells are J-chain negative. They often show strong cytoplasmic staining for immunoglobulin heavy and light chains, but this is due to uptake by the cell, rather than synthesis. The inability of H/RS cells to synthesize immunoglobulin has been attributed to defective gene transcription. The transcription factors BOB-1 and Oct-2, found in normal B-cells, may be expressed individually in H/RS cells, but it is claimed that they do not occur together. B-cell specific activation protein (BSAP; a product of the *PAX5* gene) is weakly expressed in H/RS cells. Gene expression profiles of HL cell lines have shown down-regulation of genes affecting multiple components of signalling pathways active in B-cells (Schwering *et al.* 2003).

Very rare examples of H/RS cell that express T-cell antigens have been reported. Despite their T-cell antigens, these cells have been shown to have clonal immunoglobulin gene rearrangements. A recent study from Japan reported that, in almost 10 per cent of cases of HL, the H/RS cells expressed follicular dendritic cell markers and showed germline T-cell receptor and immunoglobulin genes (Nakamura *et al.* 1999). Thus, it appears that, while the majority of cases of CHL have H/RS cells of B-cell origin, a minority of cases may have a different histogenesis. Almost all H/RS cells show positive staining for Ki67 and thus appear to be in cycle.

GENETICS

The large majority of CHL cases studied have shown monoclonal immunoglobulin gene rearrangements. The variable region genes show a high degree of intraclonal mutations characteristic of germinal centre B-cells. Very few cases of CHL in which the H/RS cells show clonal T-cell gene rearrangements have been observed. Conventional cytogenetics, fluorescence *in-situ* hybridization (FISH) and comparative genomic hybridization have shown aneuploidy in H/RS cells, but no specific chromosomal abnormality has been identified.

EPSTEIN–BARR VIRUS

Latent EBV infection is found in a proportion of patients with CHL. The H/RS cells in these cases contain EBERs

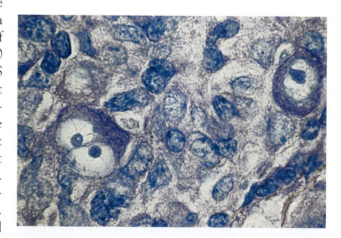

FIGURE 8.6 Giemsa-stained section of classical Hodgkin lymphoma showing a Reed–Sternberg cell and a mononuclear Hodgkin cell. Both cell show deep cytoplasmic basophilia.

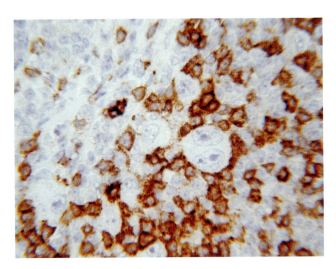

FIGURE 8.7 Classic Hodgkin lymphoma stained for CD3. T-Cells are the predominant cell type and show tight rosetting of a Reed–Sternberg cell.

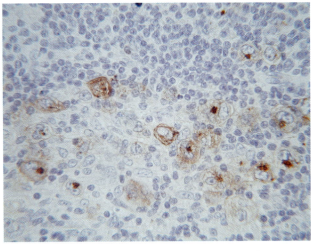

FIGURE 8.9 Classic Hodgkin lymphoma stained for CD15. Note the membrane and cytoplasmic staining with Golgi zone accentuation in this case.

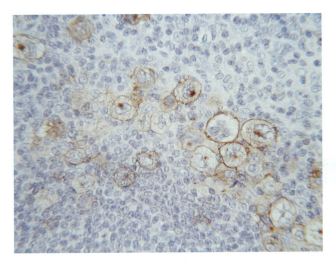

FIGURE 8.8 Classic Hodgkin lymphoma stained for CD30. Note the strong positive staining of the cell membrane and Golgi region.

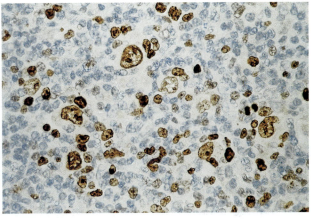

FIGURE 8.10 Classical Hodgkin lymphoma stained for Ki67. All Hodgkin/Reed–Sternberg cells are in cycle and show positive nuclear staining. The nuclei of these cells are recognizable by their large size.

and express latent membrane protein-1 (LMP-1) and EBNA1 (latency pattern II). EBER-positive small lymphocytes may be present in cases in which the H/RS cells are negative. The incidence of EBV latency in H/RS cells is highest in patients with acquired immune deficiency syndrome (AIDS)-related CHL (90 per cent) and in mixed-cellularity CHL (70 per cent), and lowest in nodular sclerosing CHL (10–40 per cent).

NODULAR SCLEROSIS CLASSICAL HODGKIN LYMPHOMA

Nodular sclerosis classical Hodgkin lymphoma (NSCHL) is the commonest subtype of CHL, accounting for 70 per cent of cases in developed countries. It shows an equal sex incidence, in contrast with other subtypes of CHL, which show a male predominance.

The WHO classification defines NSCHL as a subtype of CHL with lacunar-type H/RS cells and with collagen bands that surround at least one nodule. Lacunar H/RS cells, as seen in imprint cytology and in electron micrographs, have abundant, clear, organelle-poor cytoplasm. In histological sections of formalin-fixed tissues, this cytoplasm shrinks and retracts, leaving the H/RS cell in a clear space, a feature that gives rise to the term lacunar cell. The nuclei of these cells may show considerable morphological variation. They often have numerous nuclear lobes with finer chromatin and smaller nucleoli than those of classic H/RS cells. They have the same immunohistochemical profile as classic H/RS cells. For many years it was a dogma that classical binucleate H/RS cells as well as lacunar-type H/RS cells must be seen before making a diagnosis of NSCHL. It is now accepted that cells with the morphology and immunophenotype of lacunar H/RS cells in an appropriate cellular background are in themselves diagnostic of NSCHL. In some cases of NSCHL, the lacunar H/RS cells may form syncytial sheets, sometimes with central areas of necrosis.

Occasional biopsies will be seen in which there are lacunar cells, but in which there is little or no sclerosis. It has been proposed that these should be designated as cellular-phase NSCHL. Support for this designation come from the observation that some patients with cellular-phase NSCHL are found to have

banded sclerosis in subsequent biopsies. The WHO demand for at least one nodule surrounded by collagen bands would place cellular phase NSCHL into the category of mixed cellularity CHL.

GRADING

The British National Lymphoma Investigation (BNLI) introduced a grading system that divided NSCHL into Grade 1, in which 75 per cent or more of the nodules show scattered H/RS cells in a lymphocyte-rich, mixed cellular or fibrohistiocytic background, and Grade 2, in which 25 per cent or more of the nodules showed H/RS cells in sheets, showing pleomorphism and associated with lymphocyte depletion. These grades appeared to predict substantial survival differences. However, subsequent studies showed that these survival differences were eliminated, for all except those with advanced stage disease, if all patients were given optimal treatment. A recent study of 965 patients with NSCHL, all of whom had been staged and treated using rigorous protocols, was published by the German Hodgkin Lymphoma Study Group (von Wasielewski et al. 2003). They found that a new grading based on eosinophilia, lymphocyte depletion and atypia of the

---

▲ BOX 8.5: Nodular sclerosis classical Hodgkin lymphoma: clinical features

- ▲ Median age 28 years
- ▲ Equal sex incidence
- ▲ Mediastinal involvement common
- ▲ Most patients present with Stage I or II disease

● BOX 8.6: Nodular sclerosis classical Hodgkin lymphoma: morphology

- Classic and/or lacunar Hodgkin/Reed–Sternberg cells
- Nodular growth pattern

- Collagen bands (surround at least one nodule)
- Lacunar cells may form syncytial aggregates, which may show central necrosis

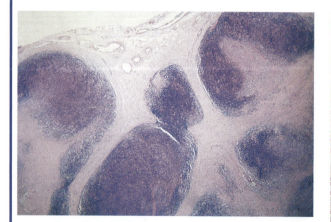

FIGURE 8.11 Low-power view of a section of nodular sclerosing Hodgkin lymphoma showing nodular growth pattern and banded sclerosis.

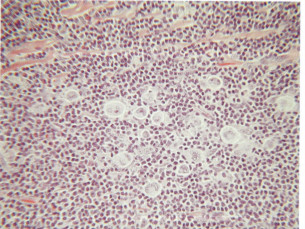

FIGURE 8.12 Nodular sclerosing Hodgkin lymphoma showing characteristic lacunar cells. Note collagen fibres at top of picture and the absence of classic Reed–Sternberg cells.

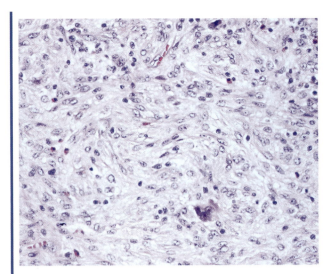

FIGURE 8.13 Hodgkin lymphoma nodular sclerosing subtype, fibrohistiocytic variant. Degenerate Hodgkin/Reed–Sternberg cells are seen in a background of spindle-shaped histiocytes and scattered eosinophils with few small lymphocytes.

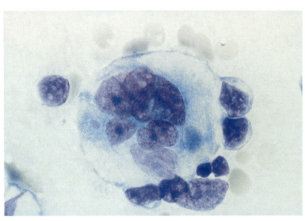

FIGURE 8.14 Imprint preparation of nodular sclerosing Hodgkin lymphoma showing a lacunar Hodgkin/Reed–Sternberg cell. Note the abundant pale staining cytoplasm, multilobed nucleus and small nucleoli. Rosetting lymphocytes can be seen adhering to the cell membrane.

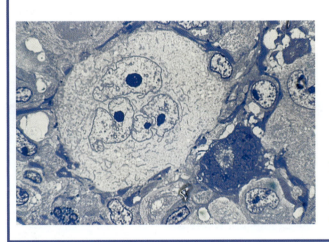

FIGURE 8.15 Plastic-embedded section of nodular sclerosing Hodgkin lymphoma showing a lacunar Hodgkin/Reed–Sternberg cell. The cytoplasm of this cell is relatively abundant and contains few organelles.

H/RS cells gave a significant indication of prognosis in intermediate and advanced stage disease. There was no difference in progression-free survival or overall survival between patients with only one risk factor (78 per cent), and those with two (19 per cent) or three (3 per cent) risk factors. In this study, 50 per cent of the patients fell into the low risk and 50 per cent into the high-risk groups. The application of this grading system may

---

BOX 8.7: Prognostically adverse histological features in nodular sclerosis classical Hodgkin lymphoma

- Morphological atypia of the Hodgkin/Reed–Sternberg (H/RS) cells: >25 per cent bizarre and highly anaplastic appearing H/RS cells with pleomorphic nuclear features, hyperchromatism and highly irregular nuclear outlines

- Relative number of lymphocytes: lymphocytes <33 per cent of all cells in the whole section
- Tissue infiltration by eosinophils: eosinophils constitute more than 5 per cent of all cells in at least five high-power fields

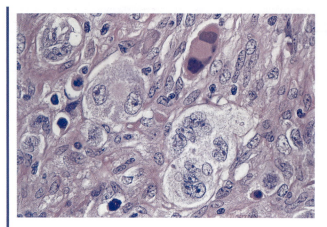

FIGURE 8.16 Section of nodular sclerosing Hodgkin lymphoma showing atypical Hodgkin/Reed–Sternberg cells.

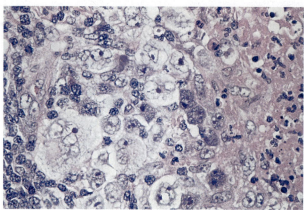

FIGURE 8.17 Section of nodular sclerosing Hodgkin lymphoma showing sheets of Hodgkin/Reed–Sternberg cells with an area of necrosis (so-called 'syncytial Hodgkin lymphoma').

help to avoid overtreatment and reduce therapy-related side effects.

MIXED CELLULARITY CLASSICAL HODGKIN LYMPHOMA

Mixed cellularity Hodgkin lymphoma (MCHL) is defined in the WHO classification as a subtype of CHL with scattered classical H/RS cells in a diffuse or vaguely nodular background of mixed inflammatory cells without nodular sclerosing fibrosis. In this definition, cellular-phase NSHL is categorized as MCHL. The border between MCHL and LDHL is usually, but not always, easily determined. MCHL comprises approximately 20 per cent of cases of CHL in the developed world. It shows a male predominance and is the subtype of CHL most commonly associated with HIV infection (Bellas *et al.* 1996).

Within the basic parameters set out in the definition, the morphology of MCHL varies considerably. The background infiltrate to the H/RS cells includes lymphocytes (mainly T-cells), plasma cells, eosinophils, neutrophils and histiocytes, but the relative proportions of these cells vary. Histiocytes may form loose epithelioid cell granulomas and may fuse to form Langhans-type giant cells. Interfollicular HL is included in the category of MCHL. In this variant, the lymph node biopsy shows prominent reactive follicles with small islands of Hodgkin lymphoma, including classic RS cells, in the interfollicular zone. It may be associated with more typical MCHL in part of the node or in other biopsies. The importance of recognizing this variant is that it should be distinguished from a purely reactive proliferation.

LYMPHOCYTE-RICH CLASSICAL HODGKIN LYMPHOMA

This subtype of CHL was described in recent years. It usually has a nodular growth pattern and in the past was often misdiagnosed as NLPHL. It accounts for approximately 5 per cent of all cases of CHL and shows a male predominance of 70 per cent. Peripheral lymphadenopathy is the most common presentation, with mediastinal involvement in 15 per cent. Most patients have Stage I or II disease.

The tumour almost always has a nodular growth pattern with small, inactive germinal centres in many of the nodules. The nodules abut each other with little interfollicular tissue. H/RS cells are scattered in the

---

▲ **BOX 8.8: Mixed cellularity Hodgkin lymphoma: clinical features**

- ▲ 70 per cent male predominance
- ▲ Associated with human immunodeficiency virus infection
- ▲ Peripheral lymphadenopathy most common presentation
- ▲ Spleen involved in 30 per cent, bone marrow in 10 per cent
- ▲ Often presents in advanced stage with B-symptoms

● BOX 8.9: Mixed cellularity Hodgkin lymphoma: morphology

- May have interfollicular growth pattern
- Hodgkin/Reed–Sternberg cells usually easy to find
- Capsule not thickened

- No banded sclerosis
- Variable background of lymphocytes (T), plasma cells, eosinophils, neutrophils and histiocytes
- Histiocytes may form loose granulomas

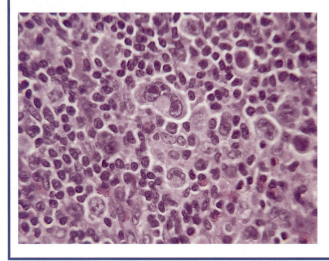

FIGURE 8.18 Mixed cellularity Hodgkin lymphoma showing a classical Reed–Sternberg (RS) cell together with Hodgkin/RS cells in a background of small lymphocytes, eosinophils and histiocytes.

mantle zone. Eosinophils and neutrophils are absent or scanty.

IMMUNOHISTOCHEMISTRY

The H/RS cells in lymphocyte-rich classic Hodgkin lymphoma (LRCHL) have the same immunophenotype as those of other classical subtypes of HL. The germinal centres in the nodules are BCL-2 negative, and contain scattered T-cells and a dendritic cell network demonstrable with CD21 and CD23. The majority of the small lymphocytes are B-cells and have the immunophenotype of mantle cells, expressing both surface IgM and IgD. As in other types of CHL, the small lymphocytes forming a rosette around the H/RS cell are mostly T-cells. In the rare diffuse forms of LRCHL, the number of background T-cells is increased.

DIFFERENTIAL DIAGNOSIS

In a recent study, 30 per cent of cases originally diagnosed as NLPHL were found to be examples of LRCHL following critical immunohistochemical evaluation (Anagnostopoulos *et al.* 2000). This almost certainly accounts for some of the cases reported as NLPHL that ran an unfavourable course, since relapsed LRCHL has

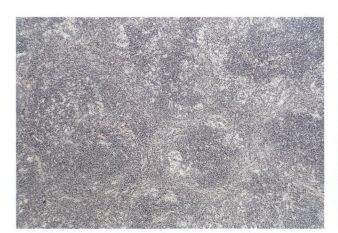

FIGURE 8.19 Lymphocyte-rich classical Hodgkin lymphoma. Low-power view showing the common nodular growth pattern.

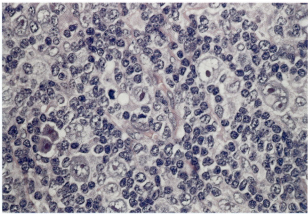

FIGURE 8.20 High-power view of lymphocyte-rich classical Hodgkin lymphoma showing a classical Reed–Sternberg cell.

a less favourable prognosis than NLPHL. The finding of the classical H/RS phenotype (CD30+, CD15+, CD20−\+, J chain−) differentiates LRCHL from NLPHL in which the L&H cells are CD30−, CD15−, CD20+, J chain+.

LYMPHOCYTE-DEPLETED CLASSICAL HODGKIN LYMPHOMA

The Lukes and Butler classification of HL recognized two forms of lymphocyte-depleted Hodgkin lymphoma (LDHL), both of which have a diffuse growth pattern. The reticular type is composed of sheets of H/RS cells with sparse lymphocytes and other reactive cells. This disease was also known in the past as Hodgkin's sarcoma. The second type was designated as diffuse fibrosis in which H/RS cells are found in a paucicellular background composed mainly of weakly eosinophilic, periodic acid–Schiff (PAS)-positive ground substance rather than mature collagen.

The advent of immunohistochemistry revealed that many cases diagnosed as reticular HL were in fact anaplastic carcinomas or NHLs that contained multinucleate cells bearing some resemblance to H/RS cells. Some cases were lymphocyte-depleted variants of NSHL.

Lymphocyte-depleted Hodgkin lymphoma is the least common subtype of CHL, although some of the AIDS-associated cases of CHL fall into this category.

Lymphocyte-depleted Hodgkin lymphoma is said to occur more frequently in abdominal organs (liver, spleen and retroperitoneal lymph nodes) than other subtypes of CHL. It frequently affects the bone marrow. Patients, therefore, often present in advanced stage and frequently have B-symptoms.

The diagnosis of LDHL is dependent on finding H/RS cells, often pleomorphic, with the classic immunophenotype in a lymphocyte-depleted background and without evidence of banded fibrosis.

▲ BOX 8.10: Lymphocyte-depleted Hodgkin lymphoma: clinical features

▲ 75 per cent male predominance
▲ Association with human immunodeficiency virus infection
▲ Relative sparing of peripheral lymph nodes
▲ Frequent involvement of abdominal organs and bone marrow
▲ Usually presents in advanced stage with B-symptoms

● BOX 8.11: Lymphocyte-depleted Hodgkin lymphoma: morphology

• Reticular form has sarcomatous appearance with many Hodgkin/Reed–Sternberg (H/RS) cells and pleomorphic forms

• Diffuse fibrosis form shows scattered H/RS cells in a paucicellular eosinophilic, periodic acid–Schiff-positive background

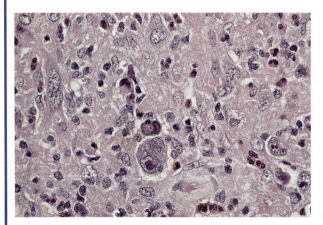

FIGURE 8.21 Hodgkin lymphoma lymphocyte-depleted subtype showing Hodgkin/Reed–Sternberg cells in a paucicellular background of amorphous eosinophilic material (previously called diffuse fibrosis).

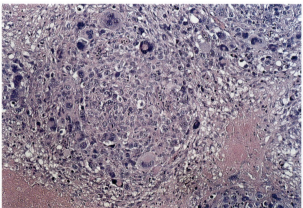

FIGURE 8.22 Hodgkin lymphoma lymphocyte-depleted subtype showing sheets of atypical Hodgkin/Reed–Sternberg cells and areas of necrosis without banded sclerosis (previously called Hodgkin sarcoma).

ASSOCIATION OF CLASSICAL HODGKIN LYMPHOMA WITH NON-HODGKIN LYMPHOMA

Classical Hodgkin lymphoma may uncommonly show synchronous or metachronous association with NHL. This association is seen most frequently with follicular lymphoma and less commonly with chronic lymphocytic leukaemia/small lymphocytic lymphoma (CLL/SLL) and diffuse large B-cell lymphoma. The H/RS cells have the morphology and immunophenotype of H/RS cells seen in CHL. They are usually surrounded by a rosette of small T-lymphocytes and associated with a mixed background infiltrate characteristic of CHL. In CLL/SLL, isolated H/RS cells are rarely encountered dispersed in a background of neoplastic small B-lymphocytes. It is debateable whether such cases should be categorized as CHL or as CLL/SLL containing H/RS cells.

Analysis of the immunoglobulin gene rearrangements in the NHL cells and in microdissected H/RS cells has shown clonal identity in most cases studied. The H/RS cells frequently show evidence of latent EBV infection. A recent report described a patient with mantle cell lymphoma (MCL) and CHL (Tinguely *et al.* 2003). Immunoglobulin gene analysis showed clonal identity between the MCL cells and the H/RS cells. Interestingly, the immunoglobulin genes in the MCL cells were unmutated, whereas those in the H/RS cells were mutated, suggesting that the progression from MCL cells (or their precursors) to H/RS cells had occurred in a germinal centre. A further point of interest in this case was the finding that one clone of the H/RS cells was EBV-positive, whereas a clone showing fewer v-gene mutations was EBV negative.

The diagnosis of CHL in association with NHL should not be equated with finding large, multinucleated CD30-positive cells, which might be indicative of high-grade transformation.

DIFFERENTIAL DIAGNOSIS OF CLASSICAL HODGKIN LYMPHOMA

Cells with the morphology and immunophenotype of classic H/RS in a background setting of one of the recognized subtypes of CHL provides a firm basis for

Table 8.1: Differentiation between classical Hodgkin lymphoma (CHL) and T/null anaplastic large cell lymphoma (ALCL)

	ALCL	CHL
Histological features		
Sinusoidal infiltration	Frequent	Rare
Perivascular infiltration	Sometimes seen	Not seen
Hallmark ALCL cells	Present	Not seen
Classic HRS cells	Very rare	Present
Cells form cohesive sheets	Usual	Rare
Cells surrounded by rosette of T-lymphocytes	Unusual	Usual
Sclerosis	Unusual	Present in NSHL
Immunophenotype		
CD45	Usually positive	Negative
CD30	Strongly positive	Positive
CD15	Rarely positive	75 per cent positive
EMA	Usually positive	Negative
CD20	Negative	Variable positivity in 20 per cent
ALK-1	60–85 per cent positive	Negative
T-cell antigens	Often positive	Negative
TIA-1, perforin, granzyme	Often positive	Rarely positive
EBV antigens	Negative	Often positive

ALK, anaplastic lymphoma kinase; EBV, Epstein–Barr virus; EMA, epithelial membrane antigen; H/RS, Hodgkin/Reed–Sternberg; NSHL, nodular sclerosing Hodgkin lymphoma; TIA, T-cell intracellular antigen.

the diagnosis of CHL. Difficulties may arise owing to the small size of the biopsy; however, even with adequate biopsies, grey areas exist between CHL and other lymphoid proliferations. Cells with the morphology of classic H/RS cells may be found in biopsies from patients with infectious mononucleosis (more commonly in the tonsil than in the lymph node). These cells may be CD30 positive but do not express CD15, and are usually found in a background of blast cells inconsistent with CHL.

The REAL classification included a provisional category of 'Hodgkin-related anaplastic large cell lymphoma' in which differentiation between these two lymphomas could not be reliably made. This category was not included in the WHO classification. Most cases that were included in this category were examples of syncytial NSHL. Separation between CHL and anaplastic large cell lymphoma can usually be made with little difficulty on the basis of their morphology and immunophenotype (Table 8.1).

Diffuse large B-cell lymphomas may contain pleomorphic cells resembling H/RS cells and these are usually CD30 positive. Such tumours have a background population of blast cells that usually strongly express B-cell antigens and are thus inconsistent with any subtype of CHL. T-cell/histiocyte-rich B-cell lymphoma may, however, have a greater resemblance to CHL. The large B-cells in a minority of these tumours may resemble H/RS cells and express CD30. They are, however, negative for CD15, and almost always express CD20 and other B-cell antigens much more strongly than is usually seen in H/RS cells.

The differentiation of NLPHL from LRCHL has already been discussed (see page 127–128). These two entities are easily confused on morphology but can usually be clearly separated with immunohistochemistry.

The increased incidence of lymphomas in primary and acquired immunodeficiency states as well as in iatrogenic immunosuppression and long-term methotrexate therapy for autoimmune disease includes Hodgkin lymphoma. In such cases, the disease is usually associated with EBV infection. A proportion of these proliferations regress when immunosuppression is reversed, suggesting that they are EBV (and possibly other virus)-driven lymphoproliferations. When appropriate, immunosuppressive drugs should be reduced or stopped for a trial period to determine whether regression will occur.

REFERENCES

Anagnostopoulos I, Hansmann M-L, Franssila K, et al. 2000 European task force lymphoma project on lymphocyte predominance Hodgkin disease: histologic and immunohistologic analysis of submitted cases reveals 2 types of Hodgkin disease with a nodular pattern and abundant lymphocytes. Blood 96: 1889–1899.

Bellas C, Santon A, Manzanal A, et al. 1996 Pathological, immunological and molecular features of Hodgkin's disease associated with HIV infection. Comparison with ordinary Hodgkin's disease. American Journal of Surgical Pathology 20: 1520–1524.

Boudova L, Torlakovic E, Delabie J, et al. 2003 Nodular lymphocyte-predominant Hodgkin lymphoma with nodules resembling T-cell/histiocyte-rich B-cell lymphoma: differential diagnosis between nodular lymphocyte-predominant Hodgkin lymphoma and T-cell/histiocyte-rich B-cell lymphoma. Blood 102: 3753–3758.

Franke S, Wlodarska I, Maes B, et al. 2002 Comparative genomic hybridization pattern distinguishes T-cell/histiocyte-rich B-cell lymphoma from nodular lymphocyte predominance Hodgkin's lymphoma. American Journal of Pathology 161: 1861–1867.

Nakamura S, Nagahama M, Kagami Y, et al. 1999 Hodgkin's disease expressing dendritic cell marker CD21 without any other B-cell marker. American Journal of Surgical Pathology 23: 363–376.

Nguyen PL, Ferry JA, Harris NL 1999 Progressive transformation of germinal centers and nodular lymphocyte predominance Hodgkin's disease. A comparative immunohistochemical study. American Journal of Surgical Pathology 23: 27–33.

Schwering I, Brauninger A, Klein U, et al. 2003 Loss of the B-lineage-specific gene expression program on Hodgkin and Reed–Sternberg cells of Hodgkin lymphoma. Blood 101: 1505–1512.

Teruya-Feldstein J, Jaffe E, Burd PR, et al. 1999 Differential chemokine expression in tissues involved by Hodgkin's disease: direct correlation of eotaxin expression and tissue eosinophilia. Blood 93: 2463–2470.

Tinguely M, Rosenquist R, Sundstrom C, et al. 2003 Analysis of a clonally related mantle cell and Hodgkin lymphoma indicates Epstein–Barr virus infection of a Hodgkin/Reed–Sternberg precursor in a germinal center. American Journal of Surgical Pathology 27: 1483–1488.

von Wasielewski S, Franklin J, Fischer R, et al. 2003 Nodular sclerosing Hodgkin disease: new grading predicts prognosis in intermediate and advanced stages. Blood 101: 4063–4069.

9 HISTIOCYTIC AND DENDRITIC CELL NEOPLASMS, MASTOCYTOSIS AND MYELOID SARCOMA

HISTIOCYTIC AND DENDRITIC CELL NEOPLASMS

The World Health Organization (WHO) classification of histiocytic and dendritic-cell neoplasms is shown in Box 9.1.

BOX 9.1: Histiocytic and dendritic-cell neoplasms: WHO classification (Jaffe et al. 2001)

Histiocytic sarcoma
Dendritic cell neoplasms
    Langerhans cell histiocytosis
    Langerhans cell sarcoma
    Interdigitating dendritic cell sarcoma/tumour
    Follicular dendritic cell sarcoma/tumour
    Dendritic cell sarcoma, not otherwise specified

These are uncommon neoplasms, often represented in the literature as small series or single case reports. Neoplasms of interdigitating dendritic cells and follicular dendritic cells are designated as 'sarcoma/tumour' to encompass the variable cytological grade and behaviour of these tumours, that is, not all are clearly sarcomatous.

The International Lymphoma Study Group (ILSG) collected 61 cases of histiocytic and dendritic cell neoplasms and subjected them to detailed morphological and immunohistochemical analysis (Pileri *et al.* 2002). They were able to categorize 57 of these cases into four groups, using a panel of six antibodies (Table 9.1). The remaining four cases were allocated to groups on the basis of light microscopical features and ultrastructural features. The cases of Langerhans cell histiocytosis included in this report are not representative of the paediatric disease since a high proportion of adult and unusual cases were selected for the study. Andriko *et al.* (1998) reported 11 cases of reticulum cell neoplasm of lymph nodes and categorized three of these as fibroblastic reticular cell tumours on the basis of their reactivity with vimentin, desmin and smooth muscle actin, and their negativity for CD21, CD35 and S100 protein.

MACROPHAGE/HISTIOCYTIC NEOPLASMS

HISTIOCYTIC SARCOMA

In the past, large B-cell lymphomas, anaplastic large cell lymphoma and enteropathy-associated T-cell lymphoma were thought to be histiocyte-derived neoplasms. The endocrine pathologist Victor E.

Table 9.1: Results from a study of 61 cases of histiocytic and dendritic cell neoplasms (Pileri *et al.* 2002)

NEOPLASM	n	CD68 (%)	LYS (%)	CD1a (%)	S100 (%)	CD21/35 (%)	MEDIAN AGE (YEARS)	DOD (%)
Histiocytic sarcoma	18	100	94	0	33	0	46	58
Langerhans cell tumour	26	96	42	100	100	0		
LCT	17			33	31			
LCS	9			41	44			
Follicular dendritic cell tumour/sarcoma	13	54	8	0	16	100	65	9
Interdigitating dendritic cell tumour/sarcoma	4	50	25	0	100	0	71	0

DOD, dead of disease; LCS, Langerhans cell sarcoma; LCT, Langerhans cell tumour; Lys, lysozyme.

Gould, lamenting the lax use of the term 'dense core granule' once said: "'Dense core granule' is the third most abused term in the English language, coming after 'histiocyte' and 'I love you'". Since the advent of immunohistochemistry and molecular techniques for identifying B- or T-cell clonality, it has become apparent that neoplasms of histiocytes are uncommon. Acute monoblastic leukaemia may exhibit solid tumours in lymph nodes or in extranodal tissues, which are differentiated from histiocytic sarcoma by the presence of diffuse bone marrow involvement.

Histiocytic sarcoma occurs at all ages but is most common in adult life. There is a rare association with mediastinal germ cell tumour where the neoplastic histiocytes are thought to be derived from pluripotential germ cells. There is also an increased incidence of histiocytic sarcoma in patients with myelodysplasia.

Approximately one-third of cases of histiocytic sarcoma present with lymphadenopathy, one-third with skin infiltrates and one-third at other extranodal sites. Systemic symptoms are common.

The tumour cells of histiocytic sarcoma are usually four times or more the size of small lymphocytes. The nuclear morphology is typically rounded with varying degrees of pleomorphism. The cytoplasm is usually abundant and, in some cases, may show vacuolation. Phagocytosis, including erythrophagocytosis by the tumour cells, has been reported, although it is often

● BOX 9.3: Histiocytic sarcoma: morphology

- Large cells
- Variable degrees of pleomorphism
- Abundant cytoplasm, may be foamy
- Phagocytosis by tumour cells may be seen
- Often resemble large B- or T-cell lymphomas

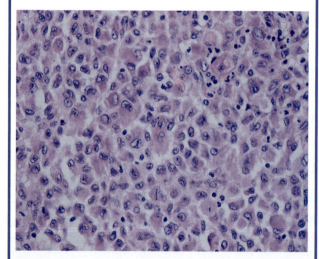

FIGURE 9.1 Histiocytic sarcoma showing tumour cells with reniform and indented/grooved nuclei and abundant eosinophilic cytoplasm.

▲ BOX 9.2: Histiocytic sarcoma: clinical features

- ▲ Occurs at all ages; most prevalent in adults
  Presenting features:
    Lymphadenopathy
    Skin tumours
    Other extranodal tumours
- ▲ Systemic symptoms common
- ▲ Rare association with mediastinal germ cell tumours
- ▲ Association with myelodysplasia

difficult to determine whether it is the neoplastic cells or benign interspersed histiocytes that show this feature.

Immunohistochemistry

Histiocytic sarcomas are usually positive for CD45 and HLA-DR (Copie-Bergman *et al.* 1998). They express CD68; PGM1 is the more specific stain, since KP1 also stains granulocytic cells. It should be remembered, however, that PGM1 also stains mast cells, synovial cells and some melanomas. CD43, CD45RO and CD4 are also expressed, which may lead to confusion with T-cell lymphoma unless more specific T-cell or histiocyte markers are used. Lysozyme (muramidase) is an excellent marker of histiocytic sarcoma, the cytoplasmic staining being finely granular with paranuclear accentuation.

Genetics

Histiocytic sarcomas show germline T-cell receptor and immunoglobulin genes.

◆ BOX 9.4: Histiocytic sarcoma: immunohistochemistry

- CD45 positive
- CD43, CD45RO, CD4 positive
- CD68 positive
- Lysozyme positive

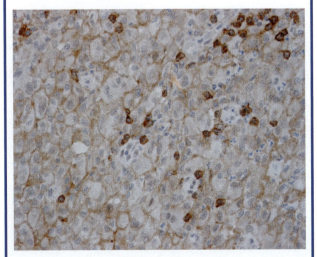

FIGURE 9.2 Histiocytic sarcoma immunostained for CD4. Note the membrane staining of the tumour cells. The darkly staining lymphocytes are helper T-cells.

Differential diagnosis

Malignant melanoma, anaplastic carcinoma and large cell lymphomas come into the differential diagnosis of histiocytic sarcoma. These can be separated by immunohistochemistry with a CD45+, CD68+, lysozyme+ profile confirming the diagnosis of histiocytic sarcoma. It should be noted that a high proportion of malignant melanomas are CD68 positive.

DENDRITIC CELL NEOPLASMS

LANGERHANS CELL HISTIOCYTOSIS

Langerhans cell histiocytosis (LCH) is an uncommon proliferation that encompasses the conditions previously designated as eosinophilic granulomas, Hand–Schuller–Christian disease and Letterer–Siwe disease. Liebermann *et al.* (1996) cast doubt on the credibility of these syndromes, other than eosinophilic granulomas, noting that the division into solitary and multicentric disease is of greater clinical significance.

Solitary lymph node involvement by LCH (eosinophilic granulomas) may occur in children and young adults. The Langerhans cells are found within the sinuses of the lymph node, in contrast with dermatopathic lymphadenopathy where Langerhans cells and interdigitating reticulum cells accumulate within the paracortex. Langerhans cells have complex nuclei, which in paraffin sections usually show one or more long nuclear folds or grooves. The cytoplasm is abundant and clear. Giant cell forms with similar nuclear characteristics may or may not be present. Similarly, eosinophils are often abundant, but are not always present. The morphological diagnosis rests on the characteristic morphology of the Langerhans cells. Like their normal counterparts the cells of LCH express S100 protein and CD1a, providing immunohistochemical confirmation of the diagnosis. This nodal form of LCH is usually self-limiting and has a good prognosis.

Some cases of LCH have been shown to be clonal, and are thus assumed to be neoplastic proliferations; however, the majority run a benign or indolent course. Rare cases of malignant LCH have been reported in which the Langerhans cells, identified by the expression of S100 and CD1a, or the presence of Birbeck granules on ultrastructural examination, show varying degrees of pleomorphism. These cases show a male predominance, are usually widely disseminated and have a poor prognosis.

Islands of Langerhans cells may be found in lymph nodes involved in Hodgkin or non-Hodgkin lymphomas. These, like the Langerhans cells that may be

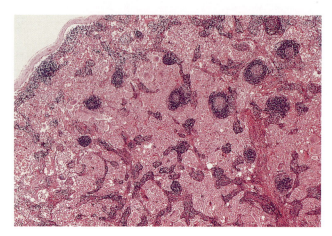

FIGURE 9.3 Langerhans cell histiocytosis of lymph node showing distension of the sinuses by Langerhans cells and giant cells.

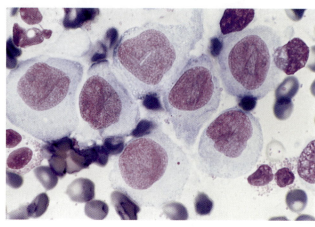

FIGURE 9.6 Imprint preparation of Langerhans cell histiocytosis of a lymph node. The Langerhans cells have grooved or folded nuclei, and abundant pale-staining cytoplasm.

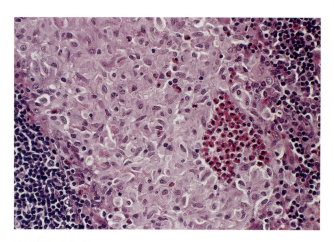

FIGURE 9.4 Langerhans cell histiocytosis of lymph node showing a sinus distended by Langerhans cells with elongated grooved nuclei and abundant pale eosinophilic cytoplasm. Eosinophils form a 'microabscess' in one area.

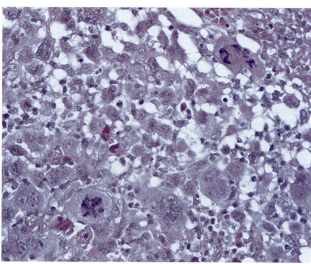

FIGURE 9.7 Langerhans cell sarcoma showing multinucleated cells and atypical mitoses with a background of more typical Langerhans cells.

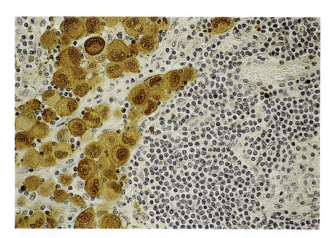

FIGURE 9.5 Langerhans histiocytosis of lymph node immunostained for S100 protein. The Langerhans cells, which have a sinusoidal distribution, are strongly stained.

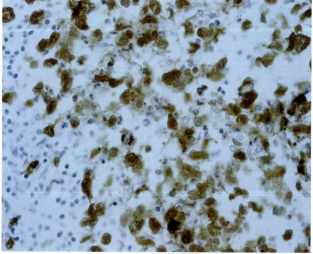

FIGURE 9.8 Langerhans cell sarcoma immunostained for S100 protein.

seen in the lungs of heavy smokers, are probably react-ive, rather than neoplastic, proliferations.

INTERDIGITATING RETICULUM CELL SARCOMA/TUMOUR

Interdigitating reticulum cell sarcoma/tumour is a rare neoplasm presenting most commonly as solitary cer-vical lymphadenopathy. Involvement of the skin and other extranodal sites has been reported. The tumour often shows a paracortical distribution in the involved node with some residual follicles. Histologically, the tumour is composed of spindle cells arranged in fas-cicles and often forming a storiform pattern. More rounded cells and varying degrees of cytological atypia may be seen. The mitotic index is usually low. Small lymphocytes, mainly of the T-cell phenotype, are pre-sent in variable numbers between the tumour cells. The tumour cells express S100 protein, but are nega-tive for CD1a and the follicular dendritic cell markers CD21, CD23 and CD35. CD68 and lysozyme expres-sion may be seen in some cases.

Interdigitating reticulum cell sarcoma/tumour may run a benign course, none of the four cases in the ILSG study died of disease, although Andriko et al. (1998) noted that, of 16 cases previously reported, seven died of wide-spread disease 1 week to 3 years after initial diagnosis.

FOLLICULAR DENDRITIC CELL SARCOMA/TUMOUR

Follicular dendritic cell sarcoma/tumour is a rare neoplasm derived from follicular dendritic cells. The tumour occurs in adults, presenting most commonly with cervical lymphadenopathy. There is an association with Castleman disease of the hyaline vascular type; the two diseases may occur synchronously or metachro-nously (Chan et al. 1994, Lin and Frizzera 1997).

Follicular dendritic cell sarcoma is a spindle cell tumour that forms whorls and fascicles, and often has a storiform pattern. Varying degrees of cellular pleomor-phism, sometimes associated with areas of necrosis, may be seen. These features are associated with more aggres-sive tumours (Perez-Ordonez et al. 1996). There is fre-quently a prominent infiltrate of small lymphocytes and plasma cells showing perivascular cuffing. The mitotic index and labelling index with Ki67 are usually low. Immunohistochemical staining for one or more of the follicular dendritic cell markers, CD21, CD23 and CD35, is always present. A variable number of cases express CD68 and S100 protein. Ultrastructurally desmosomes are observed between the dendritic cell processes and desmoplakin expression may be seen using immunohistochemistry on frozen sections.

Follicular dendritic cell sarcoma usually runs a vari-able course. Of 42 cases reviewed by Chan et al. (1997), seven patients died of their disease, 18 devel-oped local recurrences and ten metastatic disease.

DENDRITIC CELL SARCOMA, NOT OTHERWISE SPECIFIED

These are very rare neoplasms that can be identified with confidence only if comprehensive immunohisto-chemistry and electron microscopy are performed. No cases of this tumour were identified in the ILSG study. One case was included in the study by Andriko et al. (1998) as well as three cases of fibroblastic reticular cell tumour.

AGRANULAR CD4+, CD56+ HAEMATODERMIC NEOPLASM

This is a rare aggressive neoplasm that is designated in the WHO classification as 'blastic NK-cell neoplasm'. Patients usually present with skin plaques and nodules but half of them also have lymphadenopathy. The immunophenotype of the tumour cells is: CD3−, CD4+, CD43+, CD56+, HLA-DR+ and CD123 (IL-3 receptor) positive. Evidence suggests that these tumours are derived from plasmacytoid monocytes (Petrella et al. 2002), and that they should be catego-rized with histiocytic and dendritic cell neoplasms.

A tumour previously designated as plasmacytoid T-cell lymphoma, at a time when plasmacytoid mono-cytes were thought to be T-cells because of their CD4 positivity, appears to be a nodal manifestation of myelomonocytic leukaemia. The exact relationship between this tumour and plasmacytoid monocytes is uncertain.

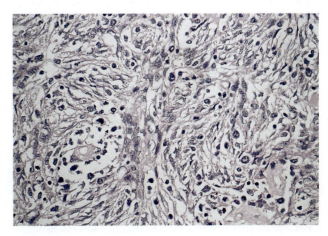

FIGURE 9.9 Follicular dendritic cell sarcoma of lymph node showing a storiform pattern of interlacing spindle cells.

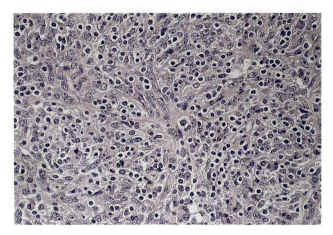

FIGURE 9.10 Follicular dendritic cell sarcoma of lymph node. In this area, the neoplastic spindle cells are interspersed by large numbers of lymphocytes.

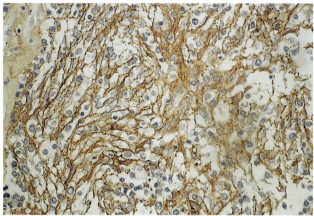

FIGURE 9.11 Follicular dendritic cell sarcoma immunostained for CD21, showing strong positivity of the spindle cells, which were also positive for CD23 and CD35.

MASTOCYTOSIS

In the WHO classification, mastocytosis is categorized as follows:

- cutaneous mastocytosis;
- indolent systemic mastocytosis;
- systemic mastocytosis with clonal, haematological, non-mast-cell lineage disease;
- aggressive systemic mastocytosis;
- mast cell leukaemia;
- mast cell sarcoma;
- extracutaneous mastocytoma.

All of these conditions are uncommon and the one most likely to be encountered with lymph node involvement is indolent systemic mastocytosis. Infiltration of the node begins in the medullary cords and spreads to the paracortex, often leaving follicles intact. The infiltrating mast cells may have rounded indented nuclei and abundant cytoplasm resembling histiocytes, or have spindle cell morphology. In haematoxylin and eosin-stained sections, the cytoplasm may appear granular or clear. If the cytoplasm is clear, the infiltrate may resemble hairy cell leukaemia or marginal zone lymphoma. Mast cell infiltrates are usually accompanied by large numbers of eosinophils and varying degrees of fibrosis. Mast cell granules are better visualized in Giemsa-stained sections. They are highlighted by metachromatic staining with toluidine blue. The naphthol ASD chloro-acetate esterase (Leder) stain gives a positive reaction with mast cells but does not distinguish them from cells of the granulocyte lineage. Immunohistochemical staining for CD68 is positive in most cases, while demonstration of mast cell tryptase provides the most reliable marker of these cells.

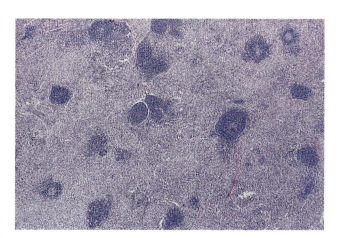

FIGURE 9.12 Systemic mastocytosis involving a lymph node and showing interfollicular spread of the mast cell infiltrate.

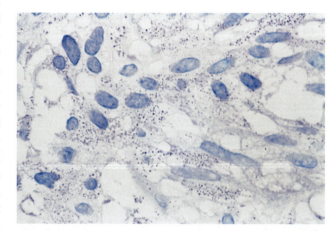

FIGURE 9.13 High-power view of systemic mastocytosis stained by toluidine blue. The mast cells have characteristic spindle cell morphology and show metachromatic granules.

MYELOID SARCOMA

The term 'myeloid sarcoma' is used in the WHO classification in preference to granulocytic sarcoma, since these neoplasms may show monocytic as well as granulocytic differentiation. The myeloperoxidase in tumours that show marked granulocytic differentiation gives the freshly sliced tumour a green coloration, a feature that gave rise to the name chloroma for these neoplasms.

Myeloid sarcoma is a relatively uncommon tumour presenting most frequently in the skeleton and lymph nodes. Tumours showing monoblastic differentiation frequently involve the skin and oral cavity.

Myeloid sarcoma is associated with acute and chronic myeloid leukaemia, myeloproliferative disorders and myelodysplasia. It may occur before there is any haematological evidence of leukaemia and, in such cases, is reported to often show long survival after local therapy. Even without therapy, there may be a long interval between the diagnosis of myeloid sarcoma and evidence of leukaemia. If myeloid sarcoma develops in patients previously treated for acute myeloid leukaemia, it is evidence of relapse.

Morphologically, myeloid sarcoma may show varying degrees of granulocytic differentiation. In lymph node biopsies, they are most often misinterpreted as non-Hodgkin lymphomas, diffuse large B-cell lymphoma (DLBCL) in particular. Clues to the diagnosis may be given by preservation of some of the underlying lymph node structure in the form of sinuses outlined

---

▲ BOX 9.5: Myeloid sarcoma: clinical features

- ▲ Occurs at all ages, including childhood
- ▲ Most commonly presents as subperiosteal tumour
- ▲ Lymphadenopathy, usually solitary
- ▲ May occur together with or precede acute or chronic myeloid leukaemia, myeloproliferative disease or myelodysplasia.
- ▲ Myeloid sarcoma in patients treated for acute myeloid leukaemia indicates relapse

---

● BOX 9.6: Myeloid sarcoma: morphology

- Some preservation of underlying nodal architecture
- Tumour cells have relatively uniform cytology, often resemble diffuse large B-cell lymphoma
- Nuclear chromatin fine, nucleoli small in less differentiated cases
- Granulocytic differentiation may be present – eosinophil myelocytes

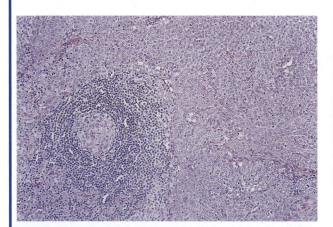

FIGURE 9.14 Myeloid sarcoma involving a lymph node showing a residual reactive follicle surrounded by a uniform infiltrate of blast cells.

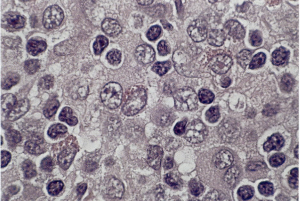

FIGURE 9.15 High-power view of myeloid sarcoma. The neoplastic cells have rounded nuclei with fine nuclear chromatin. Three cells in this photograph show eosinophilic cytoplasmic granules.

◆ **BOX 9.7: Myeloid sarcoma: immunohistochemisty**

- No reactivity with B- or T-cell lineage markers
- CD43 positivity, even in undifferentiated tumours
- CD15, myeloperoxidase and neutrophil elastase identify granulocytic differentiation

- Lysozyme and CD68 (PGM1) identify histiocytic differentiation
- CD34, CD117 (c-KIT receptor) positive

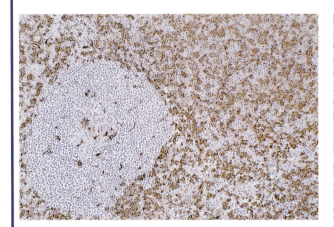

FIGURE 9.16 Myeloid sarcoma of lymph node immunostained for CD68 (PGM1) showing positivity of many of the myeloid cells surrounding a reactive follicle.

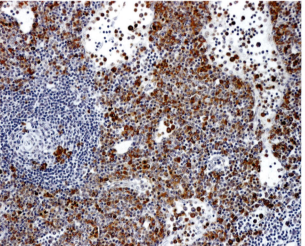

FIGURE 9.17 Myeloid sarcoma immunostained for neutrophil elastase. Many of the cells show granulocytic differentiation.

by reticulin and residual follicles. The tumour cells have rounded or indented nuclei that, in the less differentiated cases, are usually more uniform and have more delicate chromatin and smaller nucleoli than most DLBCL. The finding of granulated cells, particularly eosinophil myelocytes, provides more positive identification. Histochemical stains for myeloperoxidase and chloroacetate esterase will identify granulated cells and may be of diagnostic value.

Immunohistochemistry

Unexpected immunohistochemical staining will often be the first clue to the diagnosis of myeloid sarcoma. The tumour cells do not stain with restricted B- or T-cell lineage markers. Myeloid sarcomas showing granulocytic differentiation are the most easy to recognize. The granulated cells will give a positive reaction with CD15 and antibodies to neutrophil elastase and myeloperoxidase. Many myeloid sarcomas will stain positively for lysozyme and CD68, particularly those

of monoblastic lineage. CD43 is usually positive in myeloid sarcomas, even the least differentiated forms. The finding of a tumour that is CD43+ and CD3- should raise suspicions of myeloid sarcoma.

Genetics

Myeloid sarcoma is particularly associated with acute myeloid leukaemia exhibiting t(8;2)(q22;q22) and acute myeloid leukaemia with eosinophils exhibiting inv(16)(p13;q22) or t(16;16)(p13;q22). Acute myeloid leukaemia with 11q23 abnormalities usually shows monocytic features and is associated with monocytic sarcoma.

A rare variant of myeloid sarcoma has been described in which granulocytic precursors (usually eosinophilic) are found in a background of T-lymphoblastic lymphoma. This syndrome is associated with translocations involving chromosome region 8p11 (Inhorn *et al.* 1995). Most patients progress to acute myeloid leukaemia.

REFERENCES

Andriko J-AW, Kaldjian EP, Tsokos M, et al. 1998 Reticulum cell neoplasms of lymph nodes. A clinicopathological study of 11 cases with recognition of a new subtype derived from fibroblastic reticulum cells. *American Journal of Surgical Pathology* **22**: 1048–1058.

Chan JK, Tsang WY, Ng CS 1994 Follicular dendritic cell tumor and vascular neoplasm complicating hyaline-vascular Castleman's disease. *American Journal of Surgical Pathology* **18**: 517–525.

Chan JKC, Fletcher CDM, Nayler SJ, Cooper K 1997 Follicular dendritic cell sarcoma: clinicopathological analysis of 17 cases suggesting a malignant potential higher than currently recognized. *Cancer* **79**: 294–313.

Copie-Bergman C, Wotherspoon AC, Norton AJ, et al. 1998 True Histiocytic Lymphoma. A morphological, immunohistochemical and molecular genetic study of 13 cases. *American Journal of Surgical Pathology* **22**: 1386–1392.

Inhorn RC, Aster JC, Roach SA, et al. 1995 A syndrome of lymphoblastic lymphoma, eosinophilia and myeloid hyperplasia/malignancy associated with a t(8;13)(p11;q11): description of a distinctive clinicopathological entity. *Blood* **85**: 1881–1887.

Jaffe ES, Harris NL, Stein H, Vardiman JW 2001 *Pathology and Genetics of Tumours of Haematopoietic and Lymphoid Tissues*. Lyon: IARC Press.

Liebermann PH, Jones CR, Steinman RM, et al. 1996 Langerhans cell (eosinophilic) granulomatosis. A clinicopathological study encompassing 50 years. *American Journal of Surgical Pathology* **20**: 519–552.

Lin O, Frizzera G 1997 Angiomyoid and follicular dendritic cell proliferative lesions in Castleman's disease of hyaline vascular type: a study of 10 cases. *American Journal of Surgical Pathology* **21**: 1295–1306.

Perez-Ordonez B, Erlandson RA, Rosai J 1996 Follicular dendritic cell tumor. Report of 13 additional cases of a distinctive entity. *American Journal of Surgical Pathology* **20**: 944–955.

Petrella T, Comeau MR, Maynadie M, et al. 2002 'Agranular CD4+ CD56+ hematodermic neoplasm' (blastic NK-cell lymphoma) originates from a population of CD56+ precursor cells related to plasmacytoid monocytes. *American Journal of Surgical Pathology* **26**: 852–862.

Pileri SA, Grogan TM, Harris NL 2002 Tumours of histiocytes and accessory dendritic cells: an immunohistochemical approach to classification from the International Lymphoma Study Group bases on 61 cases. *Histopathology* **41**: 1–29.

METASTATIC CARCINOMAS AND MELANOMAS

A number of non-haematolymphoid proliferations cause lymphadenopathy that may clinically simulate malignant lymphoma. The commonest of these are metastatic anaplastic carcinomas and melanomas, which may mimic large cell lymphomas and occasionally Hodgkin lymphoma. Carcinomas usually have a more cohesive growth pattern than malignant lymphomas and, in their early stages, may be predominantly sinusoidal in their distribution. However, sinusoidal distribution is also seen in some cases of anaplastic large cell lymphoma and diffuse large B-cell lymphomas. Although an important and sometimes difficult differential diagnosis in the past, the distinction between metastatic tumours and malignant lymphomas is now readily made using immunohistochemistry. Now that lymphoma subtypes have been more precisely identified and their morphological features defined, it is usually possible to differentiate between metastatic tumours and malignant lymphomas on cytomorphology alone in good-quality histological sections.

SPINDLE CELL NEOPLASMS/ PROLIFERATIONS

Rare spindle cell neoplasms/proliferations may cause lymphadenopathy (usually solitary). These are readily distinguished histologically from malignant lymphomas, although they may bear some resemblance to dendritic cell neoplasms.

Palisaded spindle cell tumour with amianthoid fibres (palisaded myofibroblastoma) is an uncommon benign neoplasm occurring most commonly in the inguinal nodes.

The term amianthoid means 'having the appearance of asbestos'.

Extensive smooth muscle proliferation is occasionally seen, particularly in the hilum of the lymph node. This smooth muscle is probably of blood vessel origin and the lesion may be vascular.

Lymphangiomyomatosis may involve lymph nodes, but pulmonary involvement and other manifestations of the condition will usually be clinically dominant.

Leiomyomatosis is rarely encountered in the pelvic lymph nodes of females. These smooth muscle tumours probably arise within the node, although metastasis from benign fibroids has been suggested.

Inflammatory pseudotumour of lymph node resembles inflammatory pseudotumours seen elsewhere. They are composed of fibrous tissue containing variable numbers of lymphocytes, plasma cells and spindle-shaped histiocytes.

Mycobacterial spindle cell pseudotumour is composed of sheets of plump spindle cell macrophages filled with *Mycobacterium avium intracellulare*. Periodic acid–Schiff and Ziehl–Neelsen staining demonstrate these organisms. The condition is seen most commonly in patients with the acquired immune deficiency syndrome (AIDS).

VASCULAR TUMOURS/PROLIFERATIONS

Haemangiomas may occur in lymph nodes, where they are most frequently situated in the hilum.

Epithelioid haemangioma (angiolymphoid hyperplasia with eosinophilia) has been described as a cause of lymphadenopathy. It is not always easy to determine, however, whether a lesion with many lymphoid follicles has evolved *in situ* or was originally a lymph node. The lack of sinus structure in most cases would favour evolution in an extranodal site.

Bacillary angiomatosis is a vascular proliferation, usually seen in AIDS patients, caused by infection with *Bartonella henselae*. Clusters of vessels, some ectatic, are surrounded by amorphous eosinophilic or amphophilic material and neutrophils. Warthin–Starry stain shows large numbers of organisms within this amorphous material.

Kaposi sarcoma may cause multiple lymphadenopathy in children, sometimes associated with malignant lymphoma or tuberculosis in the same lymph nodes. Most such cases have been reported from southern Europe or Africa. Adult disease is seen most commonly in patients with AIDS. It occurs most frequently in the capsular or subcapsular region of the node and may be confused with vascular transformation of the sinuses. The distinguishing features of Kaposi sarcoma are fascicles of spindle cell that often contain eosinophilic hyaline globules. The tumour shows varying degrees of vascularity. Red cells are seen in non-endothelial-lined clefts between the spindle cells. Mitoses are usually easily found among the spindle cells.

EPITHELIAL AND NEURAL INCLUSIONS

Mullerian inclusions may be seen in pelvic lymph nodes in females. These glandular structures should not be misinterpreted as metastatic adenocarcinoma.

Endometriosis of pelvic lymph nodes is identified by the presence of both glandular and stromal elements.

Decidualization of lymph nodes is occasionally encountered in lymph node biopsies from pregnant women. This usually appears to be due to decidualization of resident nodal cells but in some cases may be superimposed on pre-existing endometriosis.

Salivary ducts are frequently seen within intraparotid lymph nodes and sometimes in periparotid nodes. In the presence of sialadenitis, the identification of the lymph node capsule may be necessary to distinguish between the node and the surrounding salivary tissue.

Various *neural inclusions* may be seen in lymph nodes. The most common is the presence of clusters of naevus cells in the capsule of the node. These are readily identified by morphology and immunohistochemistry.

11 NEEDLE CORE BIOPSIES OF LYMPH NODES

Since we began working on this book, we have seen a rapid increase in the use of needle core biopsies of lymph nodes for diagnostic purposes. These are often taken by radiologists using computed tomography (CT) guidance and are thus targeted at the node that appears most pathological rather than the most accessible one. CT-guided needle biopsies have been of particular value in the diagnosis of deep-seated lesions, such as retroperitoneal tumours, that would previously have required laparoscopy or laparotomy. The biopsy can be relatively easily repeated should the first one be unsatisfactory or unrepresentative. If the diagnosis is of a lymphoma, the patient can begin chemotherapy immediately without having to await recovery from abdominal surgery.

While needle core biopsies are clearly of advantage for deep-seated lesions and cases where the patient is debilitated, we have been of the opinion that superficial lymph nodes in patients who are reasonably fit should be biopsied by open surgery. However, we are now seeing increasing numbers of such cases undergoing needle core biopsy, and, in most instances, a definitive diagnosis can be made. In view of the ease and speed of needle core biopsies, it is inevitable that their use will increase, with open biopsy being reserved for those lymph nodes in which the core biopsy is inconclusive.

We have, therefore, set out in this chapter our approach to the diagnosis of needle core biopsies with illustrations of the common lymphomas encountered. The handling of needle core is described in Chapter 1. It is important that sufficient sections are cut for morphology and immunohistochemistry initially because recutting into the block usually results in the loss of tissue. Other than in exceptional circumstances it is wise to make a careful morphological assessment before ordering targeted immunohistochemistry.

The advantages of needle core biopsies are:

- they do not require inpatient admission or booking a surgeon;
- they have low morbidity;
- they are particularly useful in staging and in identifying recurrent disease;
- they can be repeated if the first biopsy is unsatisfactory or unrepresentative;
- additional cores can be taken to obtain tissue for cytogenetics, molecular biology, etc.;
- the small size of the biopsy allows rapid fixation.

The disadvantages of needle core biopsies are:

- the small size of the biopsy may make diagnosis difficult in the case of a non-homogeneous lesion;
- the small size of the biopsy may result in failure to detect variability in tumour (e.g. areas of high-grade transformation may be missed);
- unless care is taken to conserve tissue, the biopsy may be cut through before all necessary immunohistochemical stains have been completed;
- with fibrotic lesions, traction artefact can cause problems.

CASE 1: TREPHINE BIOPSY OF A RETROPERITONEAL MASS

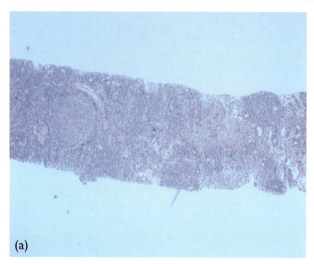

(a)

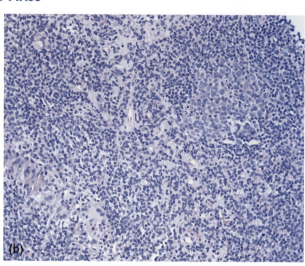

(b)

FIGURE 11.1 Trephine biopsy of a retroperitoneal mass. (a) Low-power view showing a well-defined follicle to the left and open sinuses to the right.

(b) Higher power view showing a reactive-looking follicle (right) and a loose collection of epithelioid histiocytes (low left).

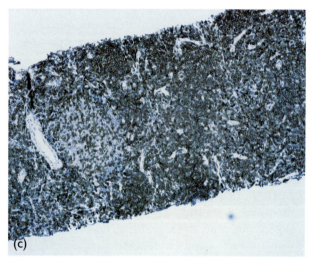

(c)

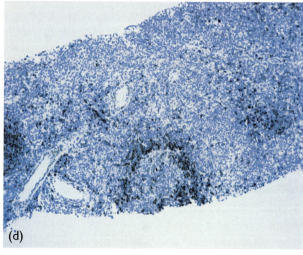

(d)

(c) Section stained for CD3 showing large numbers of T-cells, including many within a reactive follicle (left).

(d) Section stained for CD79a showing scattered B-lymphocytes and plasma cells. The mantle around a reactive follicle (centre) is well defined.

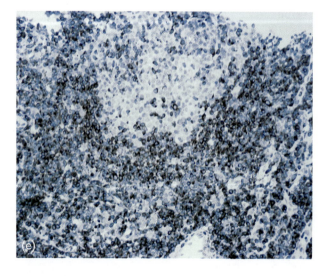

(e)

(e) Section stained for BCL-2 showing positive staining of small B- and T-cells. The follicle centre cells (upper centre) are negative.

Conclusion: The features indicate that this is a reactive lymph node and that it is presumably not representative of the retroperitoneal mass.

CASE 2: TREPHINE BIOPSY OF A CERVICAL LYMPH NODE

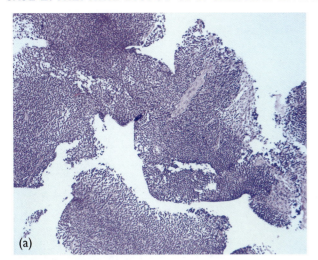

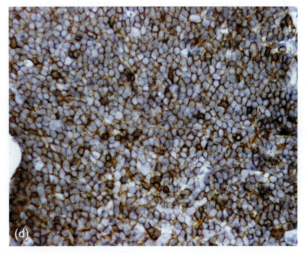

FIGURE 11.2 (a) Low-power view showing a fragmented core composed of regular small lymphoid cells.

(b) Higher power view showing regular small lymphoid cells with rounded nuclei and clumped chromatin. Occasional cells have more open chromatin and prominent central nucleoli (paraimmunoblasts).

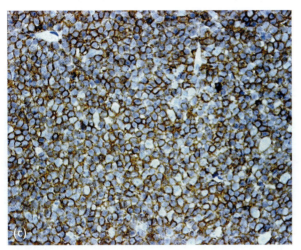

(c) Section stained for CD20 showing strong positivity of tumour cells.

(d) Section stained for CD5 showing positivity of tumour cells. The cells staining very darkly are reactive T-cells.

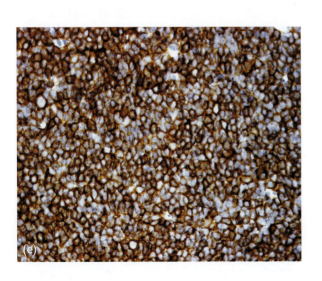

(e) Section stained for CD23. The tumour cells are strongly positive.

Conclusion: The morphological appearances and histochemical profile indicate that this is B-cell chronic lymphocytic leukaemia/small lymphocytic lymphoma (B-CLL/SLL).

CASE 3: TREPHINE BIOPSY OF AN AXILLARY LYMPH NODE

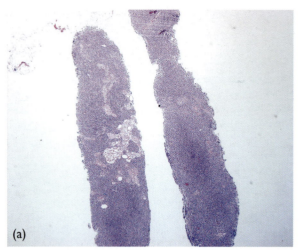

(a)

FIGURE 11.3 (a) Low-power view showing uniform dense cellularity, although the presence of open sinuses raises the possibility that this is a reactive process.

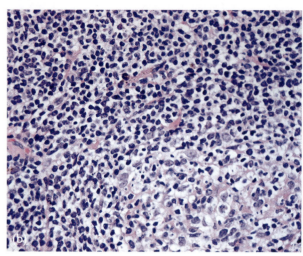

(b)

(b) High-power view showing a 'regressed' germinal centre. The surrounding small lymphoid cells have slightly angulated nuclei.

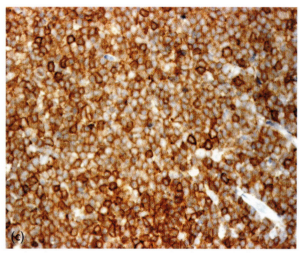

(c)

(c) Section stained for CD5 showing positivity of all the small lymphoid cells. The minority darkly staining cells are reactive T-cells. The majority of the cells were also positive for CD20 and CD79a.

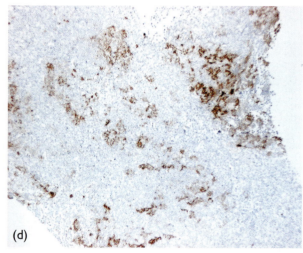

(d)

(d) Section stained for CD23, showing dispersed follicular dendritic cells. The small lymphoid cells are negative.

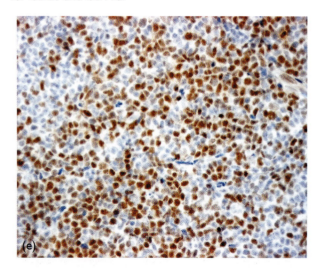

(e)

(e) Section stained for cyclin D1 (BCL-1) showing strong nuclear positivity of the tumour cells.

Conclusion: The morphological features and immunohistochemistry indicates partial involvement of the node by mantle cell lymphoma.

CASE 4: TREPHINE BIOPSY OF AN ABDOMINAL LYMPH NODE

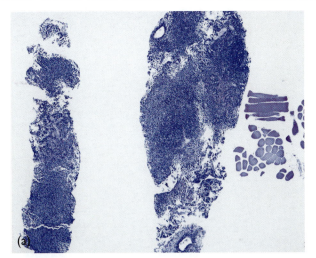

FIGURE 11.4 (a) The cores show a dense uniform infiltrate with some pink-staining areas.

(b) High-power view showing that many of the lymphoid cells have plasmacytic features. One large cell (centre left) shows prominent intranuclear inclusions.

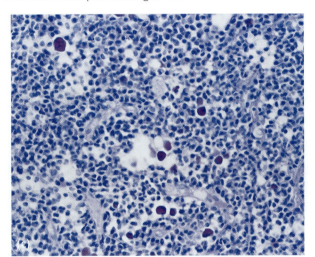

(c) Section stained by the periodic acid–Schiff (PAS) technique showing PAS-positive inclusions in many cells (Dutcher bodies).

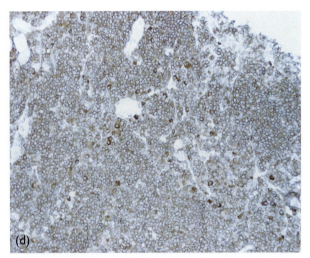

(d) Section stained for CD79a. The tumour cells are positive with the strongest positivity expressed by those showing plasmacytic differentiation.

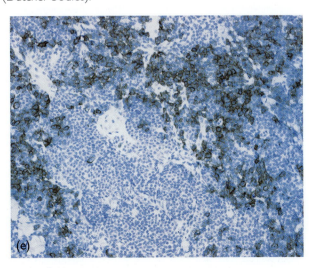

(e) Section stained for epithelioid membrane antigen (EMA) showing negativity of the lymphoid cells with strong expression of EMA on the plasmacytoid cells.

Conclusion: The appearances are those of a lymphoplasmacytic lymphoma. The plasmacytoid cells and the inclusions stained for immunoglobulin M (IgM) kappa and the patient had an IgM paraprotein (Waldenström macroglobulinaemia).

CASE 5: TREPHINE BIOPSY OF A RETROPERITONEAL MASS

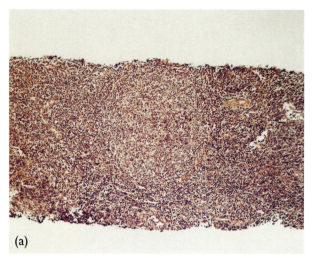

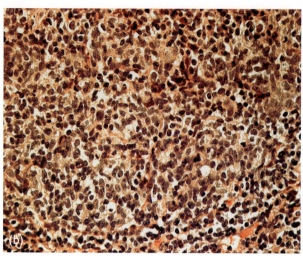

FIGURE 11.5 (a) Core biopsy showing an ill-defined folli-cle (centre).

(b) High-power view of the follicle, showing a predominance of small centrocytes with very occasional centroblasts.

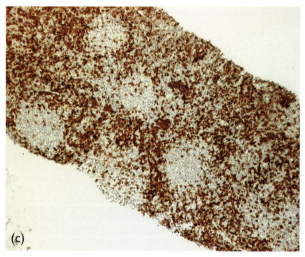

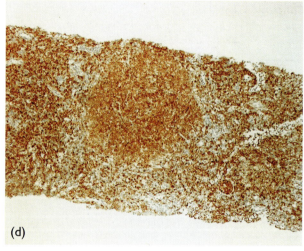

(c) Section stained for CD3 showing many T-cells that outline follicles that are not so easily defined in haematoxylin and eosin-stained sections.

(d) Section stained for CD79a shows a large follicle (centre) that lacks a rim of mantle cells.

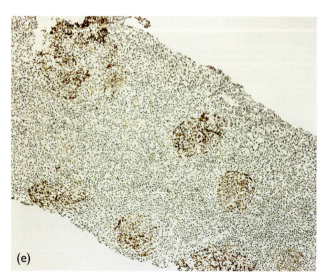

(e) Section stained for CD21 showing several slightly dispersed follicular dendritic cell networks.

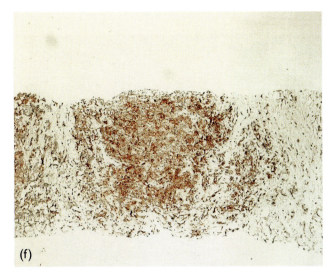

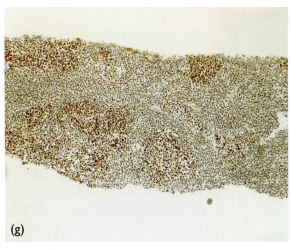

(g)

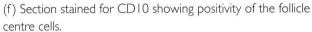

(f)

(f) Section stained for CD10 showing positivity of the follicle centre cells.

(g) Section stained for BCL-6 showing nuclear positivity of the follicle centre cells.

Conclusion: The morphology and the immunohistochemistry indicate that this is a follicle centre cell lymphoma. The follicle centre cells were BCL-2 positive. Not all the stains shown here were necessary to reach the diagnosis. They have been shown to illustrate how immunohistochemistry highlights the follicular structure that is often less easily detected in routine sections.

CASE 6: TREPHINE BIOPSY OF A RETROPERITONEAL MASS

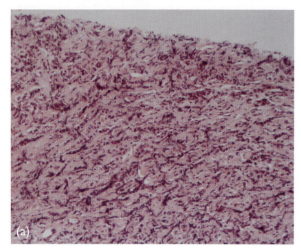

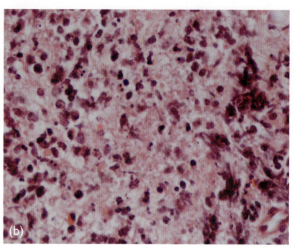

FIGURE 11.6 (a) Low-power view showing a fibrotic background with very marked traction artefact of the tumour cells.

(b) High-power view showing occasional large cells with rounded nuclei, necrotic debris and apoptotic fragments together with cells showing traction artefact.

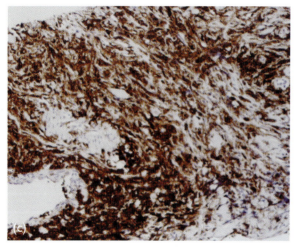

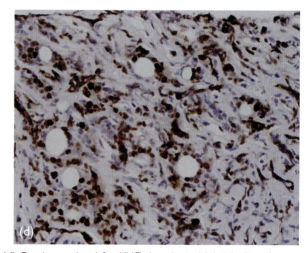

(c) Section stained for CD20 showing strong positivity of the tumour cells.

(d) Section stained for Ki67 showing a high labelling fraction amongst rounded and distorted tumour cell nuclei.

Conclusion: This biopsy shows severe traction artefact. The presence of occasional clusters of rounded nuclei and of apoptotic fragments is consistent with a large B-cell lymphoma. The expression of B-cell antigens and the high labelling fraction with Ki67 supports this diagnosis.

CASE 7: TREPHINE BIOPSY OF A MEDIASTINAL MASS

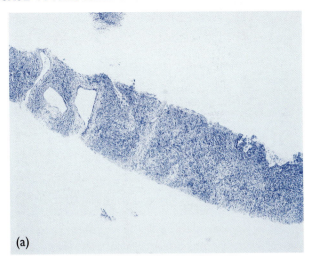

(a)

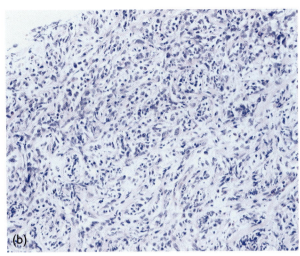

(b)

FIGURE 11.7 (a) Low-power view showing a diffuse fibrotic background with some residual airway structures (left).

(b) Medium power view showing large cells, scattered apoptotic fragments and occasional eosinophils. There is a diffuse fibrotic background.

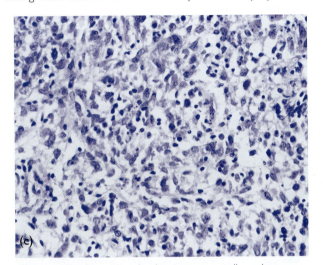

(c)

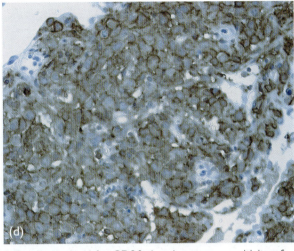

(d)

(c) High-power view showing large tumour cells and numerous apoptotic bodies.

(d) Section stained for CD20 showing strong positivity of the tumour cells.

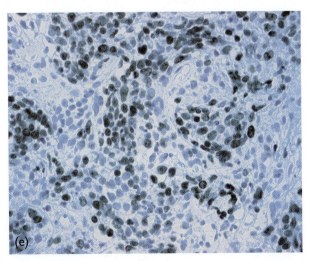

(e)

(e) Section stained for Ki67 showing a high labelling fraction of the tumour cells.

Conclusion: The morphology is that of a mediastinal diffuse large B-cell lymphoma. Immunohistochemical staining supports this diagnosis.

CASE 8: TREPHINE BIOPSY OF AN ABDOMINAL MASS

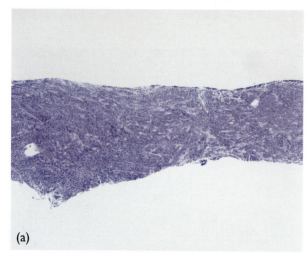

(a)

FIGURE 11.8 (a) Low-power view showing a core of highly cellular tumour with a diffuse growth pattern.

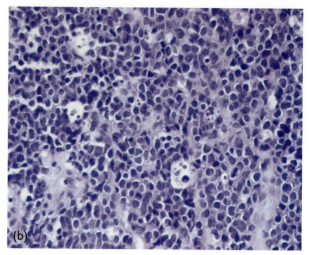

(b)

(b) High-power view shows a diffuse neoplasm of medium-sized cells with smooth nuclear chromatin and inconspicuous nucleoli. Occasional mitotic figures are seen. Apoptotic bodies are present between the tumour cells and within 'starry-sky' macrophages.

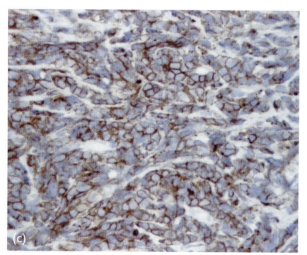

(c)

(c) Section stained for CD10 showing positivity of the tumour cells. They were also positive for CD20 and Cd79a.

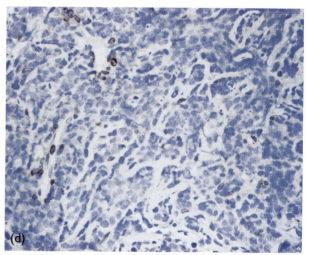

(d)

(d) Section stained for BCL-2. The tumour cells are negative. Occasional reactive T-cells show cytoplasmic positivity.

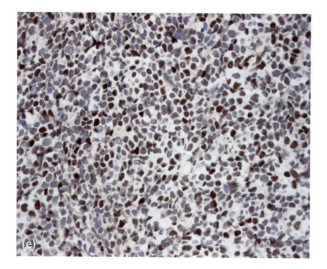

(e)

(e) Section stained for BCL-6 showing strong nuclear positivity of the tumour cells.

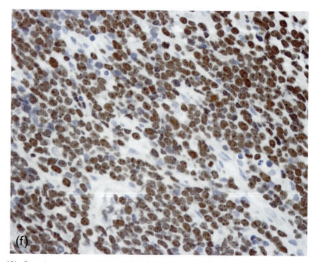

(f)

(f) Section stained for Ki67 showing a labelling fraction in the region of 100 per cent.

Conclusion: The morphology and immunohistochemistry support a diagnosis of Burkitt lymphoma.

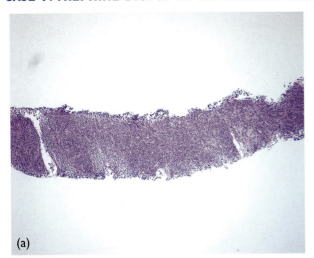

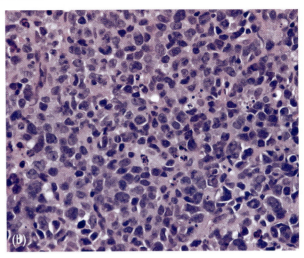

FIGURE 11.9 (a) Low-power view of the core biopsy showing a highly cellular diffuse neoplasm.

(b) High-power view showing a large cell lymphoma. Many of the tumour cells have indented or folded nuclei with fine chromatin and one or more eosinophilic nuclei. Numerous apoptotic bodies are seen.

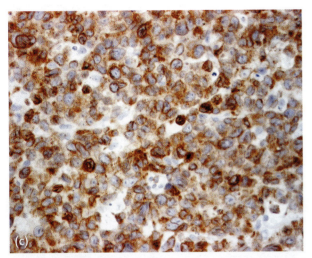

(c) Section stained for CD3 showing strong cytoplasmic positivity of the tumour cells.

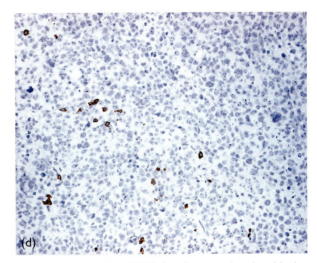

(d) Section stained for CD20 showing occasional residual small B-cells. The tumour cells are negative, although some show nucleolar staining.

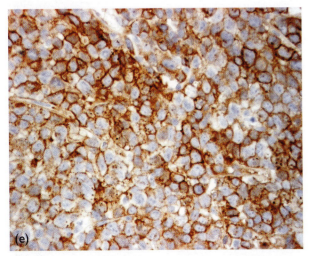

(e) Section stained for CD30 showing strong positivity of the tumour cells.

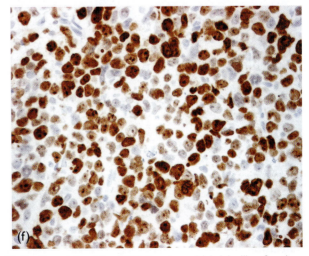

(f) Section stained for Ki67 showing a high labelling fraction.

Conclusion: The morphology and immunohistochemistry supports the diagnosis of a peripheral T-cell lymphoma NOS. The tumour is CD30 positive but does not have the morphology of an anaplastic large cell lymphoma and was ALK-1 negative.

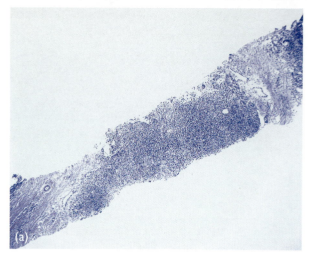

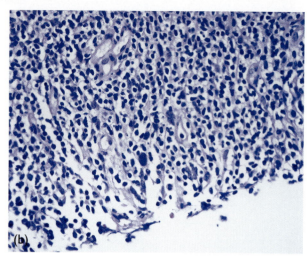

FIGURE 11.10 (a) Low-power view of the core biopsy showing two areas of banded sclerosis separating a lymphoid proliferation.

(b) High-power view showing predominantly small lymphocytes with occasional cell with large irregular nuclei (lower centre).

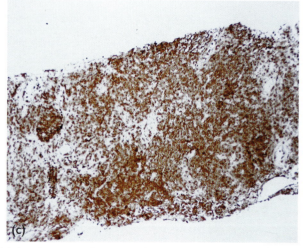

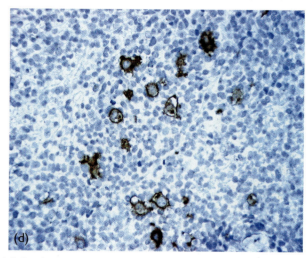

(c) Section stained for CD3 showing that the majority of the small lymphocytes present are T-cells.

(d) Section stained for CD30. Several large cells showing positive staining of the cell membrane and Golgi region are seen. Several of these cells have prominent nucleoli but none resemble classic Hodgkin/Reed–Sternberg (H/RS) cells.

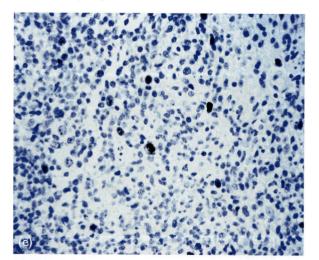

(e) Section stained for Ki67 showing that the large cells are in cycle.

Conclusion: The site, morphology and immunohistochemistry of this tumour are suggestive of Hodgkin lymphoma. However, the large cells are not surrounded by a rosette of T-cells, and cells with the morphology of Hodgkin/Reed–Sternberg cells are not seen. Such a case can only be resolved by taking into account all clinical and radiological features. A repeat biopsy might be the appropriate way forward.

INDEX